WHAT NURSES KNOW...

GLUTEN−FREE
LIFESTYLE

WHAT NURSES KNOW ...

GLUTEN-FREE
LIFESTYLE

Sylvia Llewelyn Bower, RN

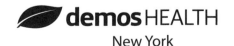

demos HEALTH

New York

ISBN: 978-1-936303-07-6
E-ISBN: 978-1-617050-87-9
Visit our web site at www.demoshealth.com

Acquisitions Editor: Noreen Henson
Cover Design: Steve Pisano
Compositor: NewGen
Printer: Hamilton Printing

Medical information provided by Demos Health, in the absence of a visit with a health-care professional, must be considered as an educational service only. This book is not designed to replace a physician's independent judgment about the appropriateness or risks of a procedure or therapy for a given patient. Our purpose is to provide you with information that will help you make your own healthcare decisions.

The information and opinions provided here are believed to be accurate and sound, based on the best judgment available to the authors, editors, and publisher, but readers who fail to consult appropriate health authorities assume the risk of any injuries. The publisher is not responsible for errors or omissions. The editors and publisher welcome any reader to report to the publisher any discrepancies or inaccuracies noticed.

Library of Congress Cataloging-in-Publication Data

Bower, Sylvia Llewelyn.
    What nurses know—gluten-free lifestyle / Sylvia Bower.
       p. cm.–(What nurses know...)
    Includes bibliographical references.
    ISBN 978-1-936303-07-6 (pbk.)
1. Gluten-free diet—Popular works. 2. Celiac disease—Popular works. I. Title.
RM237.86.B68 2011
616.3'99—dc22   2011006014

Special discounts on bulk quantities of Demos Health books are available to corpo-rations, professional associations, pharmaceutical companies, health care organiza-tions, and other qualifying groups. For details, please contact:

Special Sales Department
Demos Medical Publishing
11 W. 42nd Street
New York, NY 10036
Phone: 800-532-8663 or 212-683-0072
Fax: 212-941-7842
E-mail: rsantana@demosmedpub.com

Made in the United States of America
11 12 13 14   5 4 3 2 1

About the Author

Sylvia Llewelyn Bower, RN was born in Dayton, Kentucky, and moved to Columbus, Ohio, where she received her education and attended Grant Hospital School of Nursing. She attended Ohio State University, Franklin University, and St Joseph's College. She is registered as an RN in Ohio, Missouri, Texas, Arizona, Tennessee, and Florida. Sylvia is the past president of Grant School of Nursing Alumni Association and former member of the Board of Trustees at Worthington Christian Village Retirement Center. Sylvia has worked as an RN for over 48 years in community-based hospitals, public health Agencies, ambulatory care, occupational health, discharge planning, and inpatient hospice care. She is also certified in Nursing Administration and Case Management.

WHAT NURSES KNOW...

Nurses hold a critical role in modern health care that goes beyond their day-to-day duties. They share more information with patients than any other provider group, and are alongside patients twenty-four hours a day, seven days a week, offering understanding of complex health issues, holistic approaches to ailments, and advice for the patient that extends to the family. Nurses themselves are a powerful tool in the healing process.

What Nurses Know gives down-to-earth information, addresses consumers as equal partners in their care, and explains clearly what readers need to know and wants to know to understand their condition and move forward with their lives.

Contents

Foreword

People with celiac disease can face many challenges in their journey to getting diagnosed. Some are given an incorrect diagnosis, while others are told there is nothing wrong. They may visit many doctor's offices before they reach the one where they are finally screened for celiac disease. Once they are diagnosed, they are faced with the lifelong challenge of maintaining a gluten-free diet. They have to learn what is gluten-free, how to get other people to understand and, in some cases, believe that they have to follow a strict diet. Sylvia Bower has put together a book that beautifully illustrates and provides solutions for these challenges.

The gluten-free diet is not just a diet, but a lifestyle. Food is necessary for survival but it is also an important part of many of social activities, including our religious practices. This book is filled with wonderful ways to take charge of the diet and make the gluten-free lifestyle fit within the needs of the person with celiac disease.

The personal stories that Sylvia has included give us real insight into the many challenges that people with celiac disease and their families face. These stories are important teaching tools for both the health professional working with patients and the person with celiac disease. The stories also illustrate how important contact with other people with celiac disease, support groups, and the support of knowledgeable health professionals are to the person with celiac disease.

Awareness of celiac disease and the gluten-free diet has improved exponentially over the past few years. There are many more gluten-free products on the market—they can now be found in almost every supermarket in the country. This book will help awareness of celiac disease continue to grow as well as help improve the lives of those with celiac disease.

—*Mary K. Sharrett, MS, RD, LD, CNSD*
Dietitian Advisor to the Gluten-Free Gang
Clinical Dietitian
Nationwide Children's Hospital
Columbus, Ohio

Preface

This book is written by an individual who has lived with celiac disease (CD) for fourteen years and has practiced nursing for over forty-five years. Immediately after being diagnosed, at age sixty, I began to read all that I could find about the condition. The first book that I wrote took about four years of gathering information. It took many hours of researching to find even basic information. There is no longer this void for information, but there still remains some confusion on the differences among CD, gluten intolerance, and gluten allergies.

CD and gluten intolerance have finally become more recognizable names in recent years. The disease and its recognition is the challenge of the next generation. The amount of research in the past ten years has certainly quadrupled. That means that there is more known about it and physicians are now starting to realize that it is really the tip of the iceberg of a group of symptoms that, prior to this, were really not dealt with.

The purpose of this book is to provide scientific, evidence-based information about CD, gluten intolerance, and gluten allergies and the differences among the three. There are first-person stories from individuals who have one of these conditions and the situations that arise around them. This helps give a realistic approach to the conditions and how others have learned to live with them. This could not have been done without the help of the Gluten-Free Gang of central Ohio, a support group made up of individuals who either have CD or gluten intolerance or have a child who has it.

It is my goal as the author to provide basic information that will give individuals and families the knowledge of how to live with the challenges of living a gluten-free lifestyle. The following chapters provide resources, general information, and personal testimonies that will encourage each reader to act in a positive manner to make gluten-free living a way of life and not a challenge.

—Sylvia Llewelyn Bower, RN

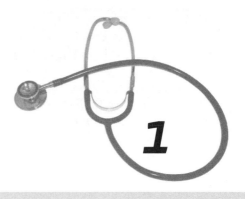

What Is Happening, and Why?

I have been ill for many years, and then last year, at the age of 75, I felt bad most of the time. I kept losing weight and had diarrhea after every meal. Nothing tasted good, I was anemic, and my weight was down to ninety-five pounds. I always loved family gatherings, and now they seemed to be a drudgery since I always left feeling sick.

I went to visit my sister's family because my niece was getting married. My niece had a friend, Sylvia, who had just published a book, she wanted me to meet. Sylvia had authored a book on celiac disease (CD), and they wondered if maybe I had this condition. Sylvia and I spent about an hour talking, and we were both convinced that I may have CD. She gave me a copy of her book. I told her I had never been tested for CD but had tested for many, many other things.

I returned to my home in Michigan and took the book to my physician. He did the antibody tests as recommended and followed it up with an endoscopy. I was diagnosed with CD.

I then knew that I had to eat gluten free for the rest of my life. My shopping habits changed because I knew that I had to read every label. My eating habits changed because I did not put anything with gluten in my mouth. Probably the last thing to change was my attitude, but after I read Sylvia's book and began educating my family, that improved considerably. My weight improved, and I was sure that my intestine was healing. My family was so supportive and was very careful whenever we got together to make sure I would have something gluten free to eat.   LILLIAN

Lillian is a typical individual with *celiac disease* (CD)—a condition in which ingestion of *gluten*, which is found in wheat, barley, and rye, can cause damage to the villi of the small intestine—whose health improves by going on a gluten-free diet. She now enjoys family gatherings because everyone knows which foods are gluten free and which are not. CD can create symptoms at any age, from an infant just starting on baby foods to an individual who is eighty or ninety years old. Lillian was seventy-five when she

What Nurses Know...

There are four types of clinical presentation in CD:

1. *Classical symptoms, which usually include diarrhea, abdominal pain, constipation, and/or anemia.*
2. *Atypical symptoms, which include neurological problems, infertility, and skin rash.*
3. *Silent celiac disease, which shows no clinical symptoms as all.*
4. *Latent symptoms, which occur later in life, and usually have no observable physical effects, and there is no intestinal damage.*

was diagnosed, and the diagnosis changed her life by allowing her to be healthy.

Many individuals in our society follow a gluten-free diet for different reasons. The three main reasons include (a) gluten sensitivity, (b) gluten intolerance, and (c) CD. Medical research shows that a gluten-free diet helps the symptoms of gluten sensitivity and gluten intolerance; however, the situation for individuals with CD is much more serious. The worst consequences for a person with CD who does not adhere to a gluten-free diet are the leaking of proteins (that are in gluten) through the wall of the small intestine. The body recognizes the leaking protein as a foreign substance and rejects it by putting out *T cells*, an action known as the *autoimmune process*. If the individual sustains damage to the small intestine, then a diagnosis of CD is made. If there is no damage, then the person is diagnosed as having either gluten intolerance or gluten sensitivity. Those who have CD are also gluten intolerant and gluten sensitive.

CD symptoms can range from mild destruction of the small intestine's villi (small, fingerlike projections that absorb the nutrients of the food that we eat) to severe destruction and/or villous atrophy (damage to the villi). Even a small amount of wheat, barley, or rye—the size of a grain of rice—can initiate the inflammation in the small intestine and begin the destruction of the villi in someone with CD.

What Nurses Know . . .

"The most common food intolerance in the world is gluten. It is found in Europe, North America, South America, Australia, North Africa, Middle East and South Asia," according to an article written by Dr. S. Accomando, in the July 2004 issue of the World Journal of Gastroenterology and Hepatology.

Some physicians, not all, are recommending a gluten-free diet for a variety of symptoms and conditions. These include fibromyalgia, Raynaud's disease, irritable bowel syndrome, and autism spectrum disorders.

CD is a multisystem condition in which the gastrointestinal tract is the major site of injury. It is one of the most underdiagnosed hereditary autoimmune diseases known, according to Dr. Peter Green in an article entitled "Cutting Through the Confusion" in the magazine *Gluten Free Living*.

You should never start a gluten-free diet without first consulting a physician, even if a friend or acquaintance is doing so to ease symptoms similar to yours. Your doctor may want to interpret the results of certain tests before starting you on such a diet. It is possible to cheat oneself out of the correct diagnosis and suffer in the end. Ten years ago, the average length of time for someone with CD to be diagnosed was about fifteen years. Doctors like to compare their patients' symptoms before and after a new process is started. Some physicians need to be encouraged to order tests, especially if they are uninformed about CD. An *immune test* can help diagnose CD. This test would evaluate the presence of antibodies for *endomysial, antigliadin,* and *tissue transglutaminase* enzymes. These enzymes are very specific and sensitive to the antibodies produced by CD. If the immune test results are negative, then gluten intolerance may be the proper diagnosis, after the doctor has evaluated the person's dietary diary. The diagnosis also may be gluten sensitivity, which also can be determined by evaluating the patient's dietary log or through an *immunoglobin E antibody test.* The most important fact to remember is not to go gluten free prior to

What Nurses Know . . .

Do not start a gluten-free diet without being tested for CD.

being tested, because this may result in an inaccurate diagnosis. A group of Mayo Clinic physicians found that some adults with CD did not always heal the mucosa in their small intestine even on a gluten-free diet. Their research suggests that adults should have additional biopsies of the small intestine after the original diagnosis. This decision would be up to the gastroenterologist following the patient's case. *Refractory CD*, in which an individual experiences persistent or recurrent malabsorptive symptoms and villous atrophy despite strict adherence to a gluten-free diet for at least six to twelve months in the absence of other causes of nonresponsive celiac disease, is occasionally seen in adults who have symptoms even though they are on a gluten-free diet. The cause of refractory CD is not known.

Jasmine is a member of the Gluten-Free Gang, a support group for individuals with CD or gluten intolerance and their family members and friends. She decided to join because she was aware of the many resources available through the group and she wanted to share those resources with others who eat gluten free. Thirteen years ago, her blood test for CD was negative, and she assumed she did not have CD. She had heard at a conference that ten percent of close relatives of persons with CD will have the disease. Because her mother has CD, Jasmine knew she could inherit the predisposition for the disease or the disease itself. Jasmine is now fifty years old and recently went to her doctor with multiple complaints of joint pain, stiffness, fatigue, and reduced stamina.

What Nurses Know...

The tTG family of enzymes throughout the body includes the following:

- *the tTG in the gut, called tTG2;*
- *the tTG in the skin, called tTG3; and*
- *the tTG in the nervous system, called tTG6.*

Her medical practitioner recommended she go on a gluten-free diet. Jasmine opted not to have further testing before starting the gluten-free diet even though it was recommended. She was working full time and writing a PhD dissertation. Everything worked out just fine for Jasmine. She reported within four days of going on the gluten-free diet that she had more energy, that she got up in the morning feeling good, and that her joints no longer hurt. Her husband of 29 years also went gluten free, so they are starting the venture together. Within seven weeks, Jasmine said she had never felt better, and so did her husband. This is an anecdotal account and not taken from scientific research, but it is difficult to argue with the advantages of a gluten-free die, because the goal of health care is for the individual to improve his or her health and feel better.

Maintaining a gluten-free diet entails learning a new way of life, a new way of shopping, a new way of preparing food, a new way of keeping one's kitchen, and a new and safe way of eating in restaurants. Starting a gluten-free diet should be taken very seriously. It has been proven that the more an individual understands all aspects of gluten-free lifestyle, the more likely it is that that person will adhere to the diet and have a more fulfilling, symptom-free life.

This book contains the most up-to-date information regarding living a gluten-free lifestyle. It was written to inform, counsel, and give an understanding of the whole story of CD, and you can be assured your life will be drastically improved if you make an honest effort to digest all the facts.

A thorough understanding of all the relevant facts is important, because family and friends must also understand them,

What Nurses Know...

IgE is an allergen-specific antibody test that can help diagnose a gluten allergy.

and the person on the gluten-free diet is the one who must disseminate the correct information. If every person does his or her part, we can all do our share to help educate the world. It is our responsibility to educate the public regarding a gluten-free lifestyle and make this lifestyle more accessible to many people who are still suffering the effects of CD.

Fifteen years ago, only a handful of people were on a gluten-free diet. It was almost impossible to find food labeled "gluten free." It was difficult to eat in restaurants because even some of the best-known chefs had never heard of a gluten-free diet. Fifteen years ago can be compared with the Middle Ages when it comes to ignorance regarding eating gluten free. Each person who needed to eat gluten free did his or her own research. Many times it was hit or miss, and many people suffered as a result. Even today, many take an individual's anecdotal information as fact, thinking that they are getting the right data. An example of this is taking as fact a person who tweets or posts on a Facebook site that they had a reaction to a specific food and that they are sure it contained gluten. Another example is the celiac listserv (http://listserv.icors.org/archives/celiac.html), which provides a wonderful way to communicate with people all over the world, but again, they are just individuals with CD who are asking questions. The answers provided may or may not be medically correct. These individuals are not physicians or researchers, and they do not represent documented information; they are just individuals with ideas and concerns. Many people might obtain information from a listserv, or elsewhere on the Internet, and make uninformed decisions that might not be in their best interest. Be very careful about obtaining information over the Internet

What Nurses Know...

The mortality rate for individuals with CD is the same as that of the normal population if a gluten-free diet is followed.

without knowing the credentials of those offering information. Fortunately, now we have much more research to give us good data and facts so that we can make better informed decisions. The people who have gone before us in the past fifteen years have made it possible for us to now see "gluten free" stamped on many products, and it is now possible to go into a few restaurants and ask for a gluten-free menu (see the Resources section at the end of this book for more information about how to obtain gluten-free products).

Individuals with CD are also gluten intolerant or gluten sensitive, and those terms are used interchangeably, but the reverse is not true. According to Dr. Peter Green, "Celiac disease is a serious medical condition that should not be self-diagnosed" (pp. 28, 29, 44). He went on to explain that "**gluten sensitivity** should be reserved for those individuals that have a **normal intestine biopsy** and a predictable and recurring set of symptoms relieved by removing gluten from the diet or a normal biopsy in the presence of positive blood tests" (pp. 28, 29, 44).

Therefore, individuals who have gluten sensitivity will have a normal intestinal biopsy but intestinal symptoms created by the ingestion of gluten (wheat, barley, and rye). An individual with a gluten allergy has symptoms that are relieved by avoiding gluten. With food intolerance, all symptoms go away when the offending food is removed. Immunoglobulin E is the antibody produced when a food allergy is present. This is the antigen that can cause a sudden allergic reaction with symptoms such as swelling of the tongue, nausea, vomiting, asthma, itching, diarrhea, respiratory distress, and possible shock. These symptoms are treated by an allergist and not usually by a gastroenterologist or a family practitioner.

Let's join hands in this learning curve and get down to some very basic material. *Gluten* derives from a Latin word meaning "glue." Wheat has two proteins, called *gliadin* and *glutenin*. The protein in rye is called *secalin*, and the protein in barley is called *hordien*; however, the protein in all three grains is considered gluten. These proteins exist conjoined with starch and endosperms.

What Nurses Know...

Wheat protein is called gliadin.
Barley protein is called hordein.
Rye protein is called secalin.

The starch is water soluble, but the gluten is not. Gluten causes the elasticity in kneaded bread and is responsible for the chewiness of bagels and pizza.

Corn and rice also contain gluten, but it is not able to pass through the wall of the small intestine. Most individuals who cannot tolerate gluten can eat corn and rice without any negative ramifications. One of the main uses of gluten, besides making bread, is as an additive in foods to give the product a higher percentage of protein and to work as filler. Most prepared food in the grocery store contains gluten, as do those in the deli department. Gluten is one of the main ingredients in substitute meat products eaten by vegans and vegetarians.

If a person is highly sensitive to gluten, the symptoms could be life threatening. Research has indicated that an amount of gluten as small as the size of a grain of rice is enough to induce inflammation of the small intestine for a person with CD. A diagnosis is challenging and does not always come easily, because many products contain wheat, and it is increasingly difficult to determine which product caused the problem. A dietary log should help solve this issue. People with CD, gluten-sensitive enteropathy, and wheat and/or gluten allergies all go to their health practitioner for help with symptoms they do not understand. The symptoms can include diarrhea, constipation, nausea, abdominal distention, abdominal pain, anemia, infertility, fatigue, mental fogginess, and other vague symptoms that are difficult for a doctor to diagnose. Child CD patients' symptoms may also include short stature, delayed puberty, a large abdomen, lactose intolerance, irritability, and abdominal pain.

The interesting fact about CD is that there are many cases with no symptoms at all. An individual may be examined for another complaint and accidentally find out he or she has CD and will show evidence of villi destruction in the small intestine. This is usually referred to as *silent CD.* As mentioned earlier, there are four types of CD, and the "rest of the iceberg" (the ninety-five percent of individuals who have not been diagnosed) will be discovered when all four types have been diagnosed. Some professionals estimate that, until now, ninety-five percent of individuals with CD have not been diagnosed.

If CD is diagnosed, then the body probably is not absorbing nutrients and is sending antibodies to fight the protein in the identified grains. This process is called an *autoimmune reaction.* The prevalence of CD is one percent of the global population. This means there are three million people in the United States with CD, but only about five percent have been diagnosed.

Individuals with gluten sensitivity have the same symptoms as persons with CD but do not have the autoimmune response that creates an inflammation of the small intestine, destruction of villi, and other systemic conditions that occur with CD.

Persons with food intolerance have sensitivity to the protein in wheat, barley, or rye that produces gastrointestinal symptoms (bloating, diarrhea, gas, and possibly abdominal pain). About ten percent of the U.S. population is sensitive to gluten. The symptoms of gluten sensitivity are similar to those of CD, which

What Nurses Know . . .

One percent of the global population has CD.
In the United States, only five percent of the one percent has been diagnosed.

indicates the importance of laboratory tests in arriving at a diagnosis. According to Amy Loelle Adams, in an article appearing in the *Gluten Intolerance Group Magazine*, food intolerance may produce hives, asthma, abdominal pain, itching, wheezing, and anaphylactic shock. Allergic reactions are often immediate, occurring within seconds, or they may occur after up to several hours.

With CD, it is important to realize that if the body is not absorbing the nutrients from the food eaten, there will be a deficiency in the things that keep the body healthy. If you are not absorbing calcium, your bones will become porous and break easily, and your teeth may have what is called *enamel hyperplasia*, very thin enamel. If you are not absorbing iron, your blood will not be able to carry the oxygen that your cells need, resulting in *anemia.* If you are a child and not absorbing your food, this will cause slow growth, malnutrition, and many other conditions. If you are not absorbing…the list of nutrients could go on and on when you consider the many vitamins and minerals necessary for a healthy body. This shows the importance of recognizing symptoms and getting a diagnosis as soon as possible.

Mary has CD and, like Jasmine, is a member of the Gluten-Free Gang. She started a Web site as a senior class project right after she was diagnosed. She is as delightful as her story:

Hello! My name is Mary, and unfortunately my story and struggle with CD is all too common. It makes me sick to think how many kids are misdiagnosed right now not knowing what is wrong with them. I was finally diagnosed about three years ago with CD, but most of my high school years were spent at home sick and not knowing why. My life as a kid was very happy. I was a funny child who was always laughing. I was determined to replace Oprah someday and have my own talk show! When I got involved with swimming I made so many friends, and that quickly became my life. Every practice was a lot of work, but I remember having a blast with my friends. My freshman year of high school is when I began to change. I suddenly was not the funny, happy girl I used to be, and my stomach was ALWAYS upset. I would go to my doctor, and I had no idea how to explain what was wrong with me other then "My stomach is always torn up and I barely have the energy to do anything." By my sophomore year I was so miserable, and my doctor asked me if I liked school. I of course said no, because I missed so much school my friends seemed to give up on me. He then told me that my stomach probably hurts and is upset because I do not like school. I spent the rest of the year in cognitive therapy working on this. Every week I would go to therapy, but I would come out of the office feeling like I was about to get sick. At this point I was so upset and depressed because I felt like a crazy person and I was too tired to deal with friends at school. That sounds horrible, I know, but I was too tired to deal with silly drama because it was not important to me. While I was sick I developed a lot of phobias, and my whole personality changed. I carried a little makeup bag filled with mints, ginger sprays, Tums, and any remedy for upset stomachs that was on the market. I literally could not leave my house without my emergency kit. I went from getting "Mary talks too much in class" to "Mary does not participate or engage in class" on my report cards. I was so afraid to do anything because I always felt like at any moment I might be sick and that would be just too embarrassing to deal with. My swim coach was upset because I would show up to practice and not be able to keep up with my group. She would yell at me and tell me not to come to practice unless I was ready to work. I was so embarrassed, because I went from a good swimmer to not being able to finish a lap. I did not know how to handle this, so I acted like I didn't care and I was just being silly and not working hard. My coach got so frustrated with me, and one day I just got out of the pool and never went back.

By the end of my junior year my family decided we needed to switch doctors. Despite what my doctor told my parents, *they knew me, and they knew I was not okay. I switched to a new doctor and told her my whole story. We had a very long appointment, and we went over my family tree and such. I happened to say, "My grandmother has some weird thing where she cannot eat bread," and I could literally see the light bulb go off in my doctor's head. She immediately tested me for CD, and in a few days I got the call [saying] I had CD. Oddly enough, I was so excited to hear this because it meant that I was not crazy and this was not in my head, and I would be feeling better soon!*

For my senior year of high school I focused on feeling better and learning everything I could about CD. I turned this into my senior project, and I created a Web site for awareness and information. I decided to stay close to home for college because I still need to work on my cooking skills and adjusting to this big lifestyle change. It took me a long time to feel comfortable eating out, and I tried to avoid any social eating events I could. It is very hard to be my age and have a normal social life. Whenever my friends want to go somewhere it always starts with dinner, and it is very annoying to try and pick a place I can eat. It is hard because a lot of people just do not understand CD, and I am learning to have a tougher shell with the insensitivity. I am not on some Hollywood diet, and it goes a lot further then just bread. I'm trying to look at it now as a change to educate people and spread awareness.

Here I am almost four years later, and I am strong and healthy. I look back on my high school years and it makes me so sad. I remember the feeling of not knowing what was wrong with me. My family and friends watched my personality change completely, and it was scary for them as well. I wish my experience with getting diagnosed was different, but I feel like it is my responsibility to get the word out about this disease. If I can help just one person not suffer so long, then I will be happy. Even though I do wish I could go have pizza with my friends and be a little more carefree, I am thankful to be healthy. My hope is for doctors to test for CD more often, and I would love to see more restaurants get on board with a gluten-free menu. In just four years I have seen major improvements, and I look forward to the day where I can be more carefree with my food choices. MARY

As Mary's personal story verifies, the necessity of education cannot be underestimated. The more information offered to the public, health care professionals, teachers, family and friends, the quicker that our society will realize that there really are three million celiacs in the United States. They need to be diagnosed and begin the journey of a gluten-free lifestyle.

What Nurses Know . . .

A CLUE TO DELAYED ONSET

People with celiac disease are born with a genetic susceptibility. So why do some individuals show no evidence of celiac disease until late in life? In the past I would have said that the disease process was probably too mild to cause symptoms early life. But now there is a different answer. It has to do with the bacteria living in the digestive tract.

These microbes, collectively known as the microbiome, may differ from person to person and from one population to another, even varying in the same individual as life progresses. Apparently, they can influence which genes in their hosts are active at any given time. Hence, a person whose immune system has managed to tolerate gluten for many years might suddenly lose tolerance if the microbiome changes in a way that causes formerly quiet susceptibility genes to become active. If this idea is correct, celiac disease might one day be prevented or treated by ingestion of selected helpful microbes or "probiotics." (Fasano, 2009, pp. 54-61)

We have traveled from Lillian's story of being older, feeling bad, and losing weight to the case of Mary, who courageously had to make some dramatic changes in high school by starting to live a gluten-free lifestyle. These are excellent examples of both sides of the spectrum. Each individual had to make her own choices about learning about CD, reading food labels, and adapting to her own environment in gluten-free living.

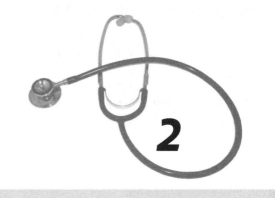

2

What Is Celiac Disease?

Growing up, I was smaller in stature than the rest of my family. I always had a "delicate" stomach, but I didn't have real problems until I was married and started having children. Each pregnancy became more difficult. I had three healthy children, but then suffered two miscarriages. My blood count was down to a 6 hemoglobin, and normal is 12 to 14. My internist diagnosed me as having colitis. I think he gave up on treating me and sent me to an endocrinologist who thought he was a psychologist. It was a horrible experience, and I never went back to him. After I moved to Michigan, my new doctor treated me for colitis as well. Finally, I made an appointment at the Cleveland Clinic with the head of hematology. He diagnosed me as having thalassemia minor (a form of anemia) since I was of Mediterranean descent. My parents were tested, but both of their results were negative. Dead end there!

A year after we moved to Columbus, Ohio, I went to a new doctor for a physical. She asked a few questions and suggested tests for celiac disease. At that point, I did show signs of osteoporosis on my bone scan. A trip to the gastroenterologist and an endoscopy later, I had my diagnosis. My health has improved, and the rest is history! SANDY

Sandy has offered her story as a way to help disseminate the history of celiac disease (CD). She is a member of and active participant in the Gluten-Free Gang, a support group based in Columbus, Ohio. Sandy's history is short and to the point, but remember that her symptoms started with her first pregnancy and continued through two more pregnancies and then through two miscarriages. When she wrote of her bad experience with a physician who treated her like a mental case, you can be sure this was very emotionally traumatic. However, it is not unusual for people participating in gluten-free groups to have been told their symptoms were psychosomatic.

Yes, Sandy's diagnosis was years in progress. After suffering for so long without any relief, she now strives to help new people in the support group, just like others helped her when she was new. She shares recipes and new products she finds, and she keeps up on the latest research. Sandy's story had a happy ending, but research into the remains of centuries-old bones reveals that at one point in time death was the only way out of suffering from CD.

Primitive people originally gathered and hunted their food. They gathered fruit and nuts and occasionally hunted for meat. The human gut, a sophisticated organ, tolerated the food antigens that had been eaten by humans for thousands of years.

One of the earliest pieces of evidence of CD was reported in the August 2010 issue of the *Clinical Journal of Gastroenterology:*

A case of a young woman [who] died in Italy during the first century AD is presented. She had short height (140 cm), clinical history of anemia, and a decreased bone mass with evidence of osteoporosis and bone fragility. The archeological

artifacts from the tomb, and the quality of the burial archi-
tecture, suggest the tomb was built for a rich person in an
area with extensive culture of wheat. The wellness of the
area is supported by the lack of other bodies found with
signs of malnutrition. Clinical presentation and the possi-
ble continuous exposure to wheat seem to suggest a case of
celiac disease. This case could be the first case of this con-
dition since the one described by Aretaeus of Cappadocia in
250 BC and could be helpful to clarify the phylogenetic tree
(the beginning) of celiac disease. (Gasbarrini et al., 2010,
pp. 502–503)

When humans learned to cultivate crops, the agricultural revolution began, and this was the beginning of allergies, food intolerance (sensitivity), and CD, according to Dr. Stefano Guandalini of the Celiac Research Center at the University of Chicago. When new food substances became popular, because of the mass production, crops were available to the rich and poor. The rich paid to have their products processed, whereas the poor learned to prepare the harvest themselves. If the poor were fortunate enough to have a farmer in the community who practiced Judaism, a corner of the crop was left standing for the poor to help themselves.

The agricultural revolution of the Neolithic period generated a whole new battery of food antigens previously unknown to man, according to Guandalini. In addition to all of the new grains, this included protein from the milk of cows, goats, and donkeys, as well as bird's eggs and, of course, the cereal grains grown in the fields. This was the beginning of wheat and dairy allergies, food intolerances, and CD.

It is interesting to note that, at present, wheat and dairy products are both listed as being two of the seven most prominent not-tolerated foods for allergies in the United States. These are still causing us more problems than most people realize, because one out of every one hundred people has CD. Only five percent of the celiac population has been diagnosed; the rest are still suffering and making frequent visit to their health care providers. Before CD was recognized and diagnosed, its mortality rate was very high, and physicians were not aware as to why. It was the autoimmune response elevating the T cells that was putting all of the celiacs at risk for cancer.

The poor, who do not have insurance or the cash to go to a physician, usually go to the emergency room for treatment only at the times of immediate crises. Emergency rooms are meant not to diagnose complicated problems but to give relief for acute conditions. After emergency room staff treat the crisis, the patient is referred to a specialist or told to go to a health care provider for a follow-up visit.

The term *celiac* is derived from the Greek word *koiliakos*, meaning "suffering of the bowel," and it was introduced in about 250 AD by Aretaeus of Cappadocia. He stated in his description of CD that there was no indication of how to treat it or what caused this disorder. He did realize that there were children who were malnourished even though they were being fed a nourishing diet. He seemed to know that CD was food related. The interesting fact is that he also recognized the conditions of diabetes and bipolar disorder.

It was not until the nineteenth century that Dr. Mathew Baillie published his observations on CD as a "chronic diarrheal disorder causing malnutrition and characterized by a gas distended abdomen." He also stated that his patients benefited from eating rice, according to Destiny Stone in an article

What Nurses Know...

"If the stomach be irretentive of food and if it pass through undigested and crude, and nothing ascents into the body, we call such persons celiacs," according to Aretaeus of Cappadocia in the second century (Guandalini, 2007, p. 1).

What Nurses Know...

The Greek term for celiac is koiliakos, which means "suffering of the bowel."

titled "National Celiac Awareness Month and History of Celiac Disease" that appeared on http://www.celiac.com.

In 1888, Dr. Samuel Gee, of the Great Ormond Street Hospital for Children in the United Kingdom, presented clinical studies of CD, including both children and adults. Gee prophetically said in his presentation that "The regulation of food is the main part of treatment. The allowance of farinaceous food (food containing starch) must be small, but if the patient can be cured at all, it must be by means of diet" (quoted by Stone, 2010).

Gee also documented improvement in a patient when introduced to a gluten-free diet and suffered a relapse when gluten was reintroduced. The information about Gee's research appeared in an article by Destiny Stone, titled "National Celiac Awareness Month and History of Celiac Disease."

A "banana diet," known as the diet for people with CD, was introduced in 1924 by Dr. Sidney Haas. He observed ten children in his practice suffering from CD. Eight of the ten went on a banana diet, and two did not. All of the children on the banana diet lived, and the two children not on the banana diet died. This treatment was accepted for several decades.

One of the big steps in CD research happened in 1953, when Dr. Willem Karel Dicke wrote his doctoral dissertation for the University of Utrecht in the Netherlands. He based his observations on the fact that the ingestion of wheat proteins, and not carbohydrates, was specifically the cause of CD.

During World War II there was a tremendous bread shortage, especially in Europe, because this is where the majority of the land fighting occurred. The health of the children with CD improved dramatically. When the Allied planes started dropping bread, these same children's health quickly deteriorated. No one dared to doubt Dicke's doctoral dissertation with this kind of evidence to back up his theory. Early studies of CD were conducted with children, but stool fat measurements documented that the condition could be recognized in adults as well.

A relationship with dermatitis herpetiformis was suggested by Samman in 1955 and established by Shuster and Marks in 1965 and 1968. This very itchy skin disorder is another manifestation of CD and is discussed further in Chapter 3.

In the mid-1960s an enteropathy strikingly similar to CD was identified in patients with dermatitis herpetiformis. This skin disorder was subsequently shown to be a manifestation of gluten-sensitive enteropathy. About the same time, adult CD was also noted to be associated with numerous neurologic disorders, including epilepsy, cerebral calcifications, and peripheral neuropathy.

In the 1980s Dr. Guandalini conducted a multicultural Italian study and found that, by following strict clinical and laboratory criteria, a correct diagnosis was reached in ninety-five percent of the patients, with only one biopsy of the small intestine done.

Prior to Guandalini's study, if a biopsy showed damage to the small intestine the patient was put on a completely gluten-free diet. If the patient went into remission and the symptoms subsided, then another biopsy would be done to see if the intestine had healed. The final phase was to introduce gluten again into the diet (called a *gluten challenge*) and do another biopsy. If this biopsy showed that the small intestine was again irritated, then

What Nurses Know...

An esophagogastroduodenoscopy, *commonly known as an EGD, is the procedure used to diagnose CD. A camera, positioned at the end of flexible tubing, reveals the mouth, esophagus, stomach, and duodenum. The tube permits a biopsy to be taken.*

the medical profession concluded that this was enough evidence to diagnose CD. This procedure was approved in 1969 by a panel of experts of the European Society for Pediatric Gastroenterology, known as ESPGHAN. This is the way CD was diagnosed for the next 20 years.

Gastroenterologist Detlef Schuppan, then at the Free University of Berlin, in Germany, discovered that the auto-antibodies of celiac patients are directed against tissue transglutaminase (an enzyme released from the intestine's cells when gluten passes into the mucosal layer). He introduced a simple blood screening test for initial diagnosis. This test was found to be about ninety-eight percent specific for CD and was quite a breakthrough, because the other antibody tests were not this specific.

In 1990, ESPGHAN published diagnostic guidelines, which stand to this day. The panel established that CD is an autoimmune disease associated with specific genes (DQ2 and DQ8), and the missing autoantigen was identified in the enzyme tissue as transglutaminase. This is the laboratory test of the biopsy taken from the small intestine that verifies the diagnosis of CD

At the turn of the twenty-first century, Dr. Margaret Shiner introduced the *jejunal biopsy*, which is done while the patient has an *endoscopy*, a procedure in which a tube is used to observe the stomach and small intestine while the patient is sedated. It was established that CD was the result of gluten; the mucosal lesions became easily identifiable by the destruction of the villi, and the intestinal biopsy became the standard diagnosis.

Just prior to the introduction of Shiner's jejunal biopsy, Dr. Alessio Fasano came to the United States from Italy. He had treated many celiacs in Italy and asked "Where are all the celiacs in the United States?" He purchased 3,500 blood samples from the American Red Cross and tested each sample for CD. He found that one in three hundred showed the antibodies present for the disease. He then challenged the international gastroenterologists to the following: find a cure for CD, find a medication to treat CD, or find a vaccine to prevent CD.

This was the wake-up call for the United States and international gastroenterologists, because it was originally taken for granted that CD was predominately a disease of European people. European physicians recognized the tendency for CD to run in families because of the evidence they observed when comparing charts from multiple generations of families they treated. Because of the constant immigration to the United States, they knew CD existed there but was not being diagnosed.

Research physicians in the United States did take up Fasano's challenge. There is still no medication on the market for CD; however, at present one is being evaluated by a drug company, not as a cure but simply to treat symptoms, and there is no vaccine. Fasano's research indicates that *zonulin*, an enzyme that, researchers hope, will close the "gates" in the small intestine to prevent the protein of the offensive grains of wheat, rye, or barley from "going through" the intestine (called *leaky gut*), is missing in the cases of celiacs who were evaluated. Alba Therapeutics is currently doing clinical trials to determine the effectiveness of a zonulin-containing drug when used on celiac patients.

People with CD represent only a fraction of those who are affected negatively by gluten. Although CD afflicts roughly one percent of the worldwide population, as many as thirty to forty percent of people may suffer from nonceliac gluten intolerance. As experts have begun to understand that this is a larger issue than they realized, the amount of research has increased phenomenally in the past few years.

A very large prevalence study found that one in one hundred and thirty three, or possibly one in each one hundred, individuals in the United States have CD, but only five percent are aware of it. When all of the celiacs, including the undiagnosed ninety-five percent, are diagnosed globally this will have a tremendous impact on the individuals, their families, society, the economy, insurance companies, and our world as a whole. It will have a remarkable effect on the health care system, because these individuals will be able to maintain a healthy lifestyle on a gluten-free diet.

Failure to identify gluten sensitivity and CD creates needless suffering and illness for millions of Americans and others around the globe. Health problems caused by gluten sensitivity cannot be treated with better medication. They can be resolved only by eliminating all of the gluten from your diet.

The diagnosis of CD is frequently delayed because the symptoms vary significantly from one person to another. An example of this is found in bowel movements: One person may have diarrhea, another may suffer from constipation, and a third may have no bowel changes. One's appetite may be increased, as in Lillian's story from Chapter 1, another person's appetite may decrease, and yet another person may have no appetite change at all. One person with CD may be overweight, another may be underweight, and a third may have no changes in the weight whatsoever. The teeth of one celiac may be in good condition; however,

What Nurses Know . . .

Ninety-five percent of celiacs in the United States are not diagnosed. The five percent who have been diagnosed represent just the tip of the iceberg.

What Nurses Know...

CD is considered a worldwide problem because prevalence studies in different countries indicate that one percent of the global population lives with the disease.

discoloration and dental defects may be found in another person with CD. Depression is commonly found in CD patients, as well as fatigue and anemia, making it necessary for a blood count. Malnutrition plays a part in mouth ulcers and muscle cramps. Some people with CD bruise easily; have hair loss, seizures, nosebleeds, and/or swelling of the abdomen; and many are lactose intolerant.

Statistics indicate that a person living with CD is more susceptible to anemia; autoimmune disorders, such as arthritis; systemic lupus erythematosus; lactose intolerance; neurological conditions; osteoporosis; osteopenia; thyroid disease; type 1 diabetes; and certain types of colon cancer. Statistics also show that individuals born with Down syndrome have a higher than average chance of having CD.

There is one group of researchers who are evaluating stem cell treatment in patients with T-cell enteropathy (inflammation of the small intestine), which is usually a result of CD. This would be encouraging, but the ideal is to not eat gluten so that T cells are not present. It is the gluten that goes through the gut and causes the enteropathy.

One can see from the numerous symptoms that many people with CD or gluten intolerance, even under the care of their medical providers, are still undiagnosed because they have not "come up" with the right group of symptoms. This is why it is very important to make a list of your symptoms before going to the doctor's office, because health care providers can diagnose patients only on the basis of the symptoms they are given.

What Nurses Know . . .

The Gluten Intolerance Group has been proactive in creating the Gluten-Free Certification Organization (GFCO), which certifies that companies have met strict requirements in processing gluten-free foods. Products that have the GFCO symbol are guaranteed gluten free.

Almost all large cities have gluten-free support groups. It would not be fair to the people active in these groups without first mentioning the fantastic job they have done, up to this point, in educating the public. They have asked the food industry to label their products "gluten free," that is, if they qualify. This is happening. There are even a few national chain restaurants that have gluten-free menus (e.g., P.F. Chang's, Outback Steakhouse, Bonefish Grill) These support groups also raise money for research and to educate the public about gluten-free diets.

There is an organization called the American Celiac Disease Alliance, which was created to represent the celiac community. They have lobbied the Food and Drug Administration in regard to product labeling and are now making an effort to get insurance companies to recognize the need for nutritional counseling after a diagnosis of CD. They comprise celiac research centers, authors, vendors of gluten-free products, and all organizations representing celiacs in the community.

Americans now spend more than $2 billion a year on gluten-free products, and finding these products is easier than ever.

The challenge is to educate patients, family and friends, physicians, and the general public about CD and gluten-free diets. It is the responsibility of the gluten-free community to help make people aware of the conditions treated by a lifelong gluten-free diet.

What Nurses Know ...

According to Dr. Alessio Fasano, "We can begin to hope that this disease, which has followed humanity from the dawn of civilization, is facing its last century on earth" (quoted in Ratner, 2010).

The most exciting event in the research world was described in the April 2010 issue of *Gluten Free Living*. The article described how Dr. Alessio Fasano, from the University of Maryland Center for Celiac Disease Research, announced on the podium in Rome at the Vatican that researchers will explore the adult intestinal stem cells to treat CD, along with Alzheimer's disease and multiple sclerosis. The consortium of researchers will include scholars from the Vatican, the International Intestinal Stem Cell Consortium, the University of Maryland School of Medicine Center for Stem Cell Biology and Regenerative Medicine, and several institutes in Italy. This could very well be the future that could make a difference for CD patients and others on gluten-free diets. Who knows just how far they will go?

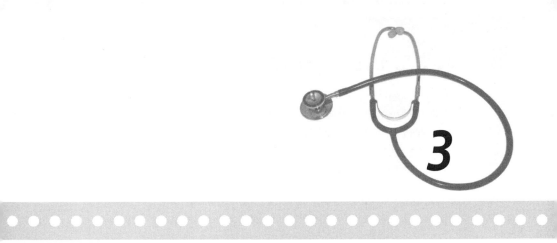

How Do You Know Whether It Is Celiac Disease or Gluten Intolerance?

I was sixty years old, a registered nurse working part time, and knew that something was wrong with my body because I had never felt so bad in my life. My symptoms included bloating, nausea, and more gas than socially acceptable and [I was] constipated most of the time. I went to my doctor because I felt so exhausted most of the time. He ordered some lab tests and some intestinal x-rays to determine what was going on. He put me on pills for reflux disease, but they did not help at all. He called me when the lab reports came back and he said that my hemoglobin was down to 10 (normal is 12-14). He thought that I was bleeding, and the x-rays were negative. I understood the anemia but was certain that I had no source of bleeding.

I then went to see the gastroenterologist for a colonoscopy. After he finished the colonoscopy, he aroused me from my "relaxed" state of light anesthesia and asked if I would permit him to do an endoscopy at that time. I told him "Sure," and so he did a biopsy of my small intestine.

The gastroenterologist prescribed iron tablets and casually said that he would call me with the results of the biopsy. I became very constipated from the iron and continued to have the nausea with an insatiable desire to continually eat because I felt anxious and it made the nausea and abdominal pain feel better.

About two months later, the doctor's partner called me and explained that I had celiac disease and my life was about to change. He described it as the most difficult diet to follow and suggested that I see a dietitian. I had lost about twenty pounds and continued to feel very weak. I immediately made an appointment with the dietitian, and she was very helpful in giving me resources. The only thing that I recalled about celiac disease were the small children who "failed to thrive." I was not familiar with any adults with celiac disease. I attended a gluten-free support group at Children's Hospital in Columbus, Ohio, and really enjoyed the fellowship and realized there were others experiencing the same thing. SYLVIA

Sylvia's case provides another example of some of the typical problems one encounters with a diagnosis of celiac disease (CD). As a registered nurse working at a hospital, she approached some of the dietitians with whom she worked about a gluten-free diet. Not one of them had ever counseled someone on undertaking a gluten-free diet. They only were aware that individuals with CD must avoid gluten in the diet.

Sylvia attended a meeting of the support group in her community, and the members discussed resources for gluten-free food, recipes, tips on traveling, and so on. Time was also reserved to discuss new products, and, of course, for fellowship. The group is very active in raising money for CD research. Eventually they

What Nurses Know...

Many insurance companies deny coverage to individuals with CD. The American Celiac Disease Alliance is working hard to encourage persons with CD and gluten intolerance to write their Congressperson to encourage coverage for this condition.

became a group chapter of the national Gluten Intolerance Group. Sylvia remains active in the group and is thankful it exists.

There are three proven scientific reasons a health care provider will put a person on a gluten-free diet: (a) gluten allergies, (b) gluten intolerance (gluten sensitivity), and (c) CD. As research continues, other reasons may arise.

In 2004, the Food and Drug Administration passed a law (the Food Allergen Labeling and Consumer Protection Act), which took effect in 2006, that requires each food distributor to include the name of eight allergens on the labels of food sold in the United States: (a) milk, (b) eggs, (c) fish, (d) crustacean shellfish, (e) tree nuts, (f) wheat, (g) peanuts, and (h) soybeans. Therefore, wheat should always be noted on the label if the product or additives contains any of the grain. Wheat is listed as one of the eight foods most likely to cause an allergy reaction, according to the Mayo Clinic, which also claims that food allergies affect approximately six to eight percent of children under three years of age, and four percent of the adult population. These statistics show that many children outgrow food allergies; however, it is not uncommon for the allergy to raise its ugly head again in adulthood. According to the Food and Drug Administration, 30,000 individuals a year are treated in emergency departments for allergies, and approximately one hundred fifty of those folks die.

"Food allergy is an immune system reaction that occurs soon after eating a certain food. Even a very small amount of allergy-causing food can trigger symptoms such as digestive problems, hives or swollen airways. In some people, a food allergy can cause severe symptoms or even a life-threatening reaction as anaphylaxis," according to the Mayo Clinic (http://www.mayoclinic.com/health/food-allergy/DS00082).

The Mayo Clinic lists the most common allergy symptoms as follows:

- Tingling in the mouth
- Hives, itching, or eczema
- Swelling of the lips, face, tongue and throat, or other parts of the body
- Wheezing, nasal congestion, or trouble breathing
- Abdominal pain, diarrhea, nausea, or vomiting

The most severe allergic reaction is anaphylaxis, which has the following symptoms:

- Constriction and tightening of airways
- A swollen throat or a lump in the throat that makes it difficult to breathe
- Shock, with a severe drop in blood pressure
- Rapid pulse
- Dizziness, lightheadedness, or loss of consciousness

The cause of a true gluten allergy is when the immune system identifies gluten as the enemy, a foreign agent behind the lines. The immune system stands at attention and releases its soldiers, the antibodies, to protect the body from these invaders. When the antibodies are released, and they go to the front line to fight, they are called *immunoglobulin.*

Gluten intolerance involves the immune system but does not stimulate the body to actually produce antibodies, making it an *autoimmune condition.* Gluten intolerance (except for people with CD) will usually permit this breach of consumption. Individuals with gluten allergies or gluten intolerance should be diagnosed, adhere to a gluten-free diet, and be monitored periodically by a physician.

Gluten intolerance or gluten sensitivity might have all of the symptoms of CD, except that the gluten will not affect the villi of the small intestine and will not interfere with absorption of nutrients. Individuals with CD are gluten intolerant, but not everyone who is gluten intolerant has CD.

Researchers in Finland who looked at children who had positive endomysial antibody (EMA) tests but had normal small intestinal villi determined that these children were gluten intolerant. Children who went gluten free showed improvement, and those on a normal diet had exacerbated symptoms. Researchers concluded that individuals who are EMA positive have a celiac-type disorder and benefit from early treatment despite having a normal small intestine.

The Gluten Intolerance Group published helpful information in understanding the differences among gluten intolerance, CD, and wheat allergy.

Gluten Intolerance versus Celiac Disease

tTG–IgA, IgG	Negative	Positive
EMA IgA–IgG	Negative	Positive
Allergy testing	No	No
Damage to intestine	Probably no	Yes
Gluten-free diet beneficial?	Yes	Yes

Note. tTG = tissue transglutaminase; IgA = immunoglobin A; IgG = immunoglobin G; EMA = Anti-endomysial antibodies.

CD, as described in the Chapter 1, is an autoimmune disease in which the proteins in wheat, barley, and rye create an inflammatory process in the small intestine, consequently destroying the *villi*, fingerlike projections designed to absorb the nutrients from the food into the body. This process is also called *enteropathy*, and it is a pathological condition.

The proteins in wheat, rye, and barley penetrate through the intestinal wall (gut) and cause many systemic problems. This process is also called *leaky gut.* According to research conducted by Sapone et al. (2010), the mucosal expression of interleukin 17A is significantly increased in CD. This phenomenon does not occur in an individual with gluten sensitivity or gluten intolerance, which is another difference between these conditions. People who are gluten intolerant (or gluten sensitive) and those who have CD both improve after a period of time going gluten free. Research shows that the older the individual is when diagnosed, the longer it takes for the symptoms to subside.

CD is a genetic condition, and all individuals will have either one or both of the following two genes: (a) HLA-DQ2 and (b) HLA-DQ8. You must have one of these genes to have the disease. What activates or triggers CD is not known, but it is thought to be an infection, environmental condition, or emotional turmoil.

Once CD is active, it can stimulate T cells that can actively cause several types of cancer, predominately T-cell lymphoma. When a gluten-free diet is not followed, the inflammation in the small intestine stimulates the T cells in the lymph system to multiply. This is a rare type of large-cell cancer that has a very high mortality rate. Researchers note that increasing CD screening will prevent this condition more than anything else.

Dr. H. J. Freeman in the *World Journal of Gastroenterology* provided the following description:

> *The mesenteric lymph node cavitation syndrome consists of central necrosis of mesenteric lymph nodes and may occur with either celiac disease or a sprue-like intestinal disease that fails to respond to a gluten-free diet. Splenic hypofunction (the spleen not functioning the way it should) may also be present. The cause is not known but its development during the clinical course of celiac disease is usually indicative of a poor prognosis for the intestinal disorder, a potential for significant complications including sepsis (a systemic blood infection) and malignancy, particularly T-cell lymphoma, and significant mortality. Modern abdominal imaging modalities may permit earlier*

detection in celiac disease so that earlier diagnosis and improved understanding of its pathogenesis (the way that the condition progresses) may result. (pp. 2991-2993)

This may seem difficult to understand, but it highlights how necessary it is for persons with CD to stay on a gluten-free diet one hundred percent of the time.

As mentioned earlier, each individual diagnosed with CD shows some degree of villi destruction in the small intestine. This destruction by inflammation process is called *enteropathy*. The villi are not able to absorb nutrients, and therefore the body suffers many abnormalities. Most people, going to the doctor for the first time, complain of gastrointestinal symptoms such as diarrhea, constipation, bloating, large amounts of gas, nausea, and abdominal pain. When the body does not absorb nutrients, to keep it healthy, all aspects of the human body are negatively affected, and good health deteriorates.

The terms *celiac disease*, *gluten intolerance*, and *gluten sensitivity* are interchangeable to a degree, but it is very important to understand the differences among them. Dr. Peter Green (2010) provided the following clarifications of the terms:

Gluten intolerance is a widely used and often misconstrued diagnostic label. By definition, if you have celiac disease, you are gluten intolerant. But it is possible to be gluten intolerant and not have celiac disease. (have no intestinal damage.). Anyone who has symptoms brought on by the ingestion of gluten that are relieved by its removal from the diet can be called gluten intolerant. Gluten sensitivity is another catchall term that is interchangeable with gluten intolerance. If you have celiac disease, you are by definition gluten sensitive. But it is often used to describe patients who do not have celiac disease. Recent studies are showing that gluten sensitivity may be much more common than previously thought. It may, in fact, be a separate disease entity that involves different organs and different mechanisms than celiac disease. While there is no doubt that the condition exists, the lack of definite criteria for a diagnosis has resulted in a skeptical attitude on the part of many doctors. (pp. 28, 29, 44)

Because CD cannot be diagnosed if the patient is on a gluten-free diet, a person experiencing symptoms should first see a physician, who can administer the tissue transglutaminase (tTG) antibody blood test.

The specificity and sensitivity of celiac blood tests was discussed by Amy Loelle Adams

If a blood test were 100% sensitive, that would mean that it is catching 100% of people with CD in its positive results.

What Nurses Know . . .

The following diagnostic antibody tests should be done when screening for CD:

- *Anti-endomysial antibodies (EMA) usually immunoglobin A (IgA) but sometimes immunoglobin G (IgG).*
  This accuracy of this test is dependent on the expertise of the person who interprets it.
- *Anti-tissue transglutaminase antibodies (tTG)*
  This test is an ELISA (enzyme-linked immunosorbent assay). It is a specific protein test. In one half of the studies that have evaluated this test, it showed a specificity of over ninety-five percent and a sensitivity of over ninety-five percent.
- *Anti-gliadin antibodies, including IgA and IgG*
  These are antibodies to the gluten molecule itself; however, the test's sensitivity and specificity are not as precise as those of the EMA and tTG tests.

The higher the sensitivity the fewer the false negatives. It is not that easy. The specificity of a CD blood test is the percentage of people who test negative for that blood test compared to the real number of people who do not have CD. All blood tests for CD involve antibodies, which are circulating parts of the immune system that match up to antigens. Antigens are usually parts of foreign material, but can sometimes be parts of one's own body, as is the case with many autoimmune diseases. Antibodies come in different classes (like IgA and IgG) which play different roles in the immune system to help rid the body of the perceived foreign invaders. IgA antibodies are not made by people with IgA deficiency, a condition sometimes associated with CD. (pp. 1, 2, 4, 5)

If the tTG and EMA tests are positive, then a follow-up with an endoscopy and a small intestine biopsy is necessary. This simple procedure is considered the gold standard for CD diagnosis. The patient is sedated and the gastroenterologist inserts a tube down the throat, through the stomach, and into the small intestine. The tube has a light and camera on it. The physician can actually see the small intestine to determine whether the villi are normal or inflamed. If inflammation is detected, a biopsy is taken and sent to a laboratory. This is a short procedure. From the time one walks into the office, fills out the paperwork, has the endoscopy, and walks out, only a few hours have elapsed. There is no discomfort, and the patient walks out like nothing ever happened. The sedation is very mild for this short test; most people do not experience any aftereffects. Because of the mild sedative, however, a driver is necessary to transport the patient home.

The diagnosis of CD can be misidentified as irritable bowel syndrome, lactose intolerance, chronic diarrhea, anemia, infertility, and several other conditions. This is why it is important to get a diagnosis as soon as possible. Doing so can prevent many of the systemic conditions associated with CD.

What Nurses Know . . .

If the laboratory tests are positive, an endoscopy is required to diagnose CD.

According to a bulletin of the Gluten Intolerance Group, other autoimmune diseases may co-occur with CD or dermatitis herpetiformis (discussed later in this chapter). These include the following:

Addison's disease (a condition that occurs when the adrenal glands do not produce enough of their hormone)

Chronic active hepatitis (inflammation of the liver)

Insulin-dependent diabetes mellitus, Type 1 Myasthenia gravis (a neuromuscular disorder)

Pernicious anemia (loss of red blood cells)

Raynaud's phenomenon (lack of blood flow to the fingers and toes)

Scleroderma (a thickening of skin and connective tissue—this is a rare condition)

Sjögren's syndrome (an autoimmune condition that creates inflammation of salivary glands, decreased eye fluids, and dry lips)

Systemic lupus erythematosis (a chronic autoimmune connective tissue disease)

Graves's disease (an overactive thyroid condition)

Hashimoto's disease (an underactive thyroid condition)

When a blood test is done, the pathologist looks for endomysial antibodies, whose enzyme is tTG. This test is about ninety-nine percent effective in diagnosing CD.

There is no medication or other treatment for CD except eating a gluten-free diet that excludes the proteins of wheat, barley, or rye for life. If an individual has CD and chooses not to go on a gluten-free diet, many complications can occur. The immune system is compromised, and the following are some of the problems that have been documented as occurring as a result of long-term, untreated CD:

- Cancer
  T-cell initiated lymphoma (described earlier in this chapter)
  Adenocarcinoma of the intestine (cancer originating in epithelial cells originating in glandular tissue)
  Esophageal cancer
- Liver disorders
  Increased liver enzymes
  Nonspecific hepatitis
  Nonalcoholic fatty liver disease
  Cholestatic liver disease

Cholestatic liver disease is the most common liver disorder among CD patients. This disease occurs when the bile duct leading from the gallbladder to the liver is suppressed and the bile does not flow.

Other conditions frequently seen with CD include

- Fibromyalgia (pain in the fibrous areas of muscles)
- Aphthous ulcers (sores in the soft mucous membranes of the mouth and tongue)
- Joint pain
- Down syndrome (It is estimated that 20% of all individuals with this condition have CD.)
- Dysrhythmia (an abnormal heart rate)
- Infertility
- Neurological symptoms
  Ataxia (loss of balance when walking)
  Attention-deficit/hyperactivity disorder
  Depression and/or anxiety (common in about 20% of CD patients)

Neuropathy (loss of nerve function)
Seizure disorders

According to Dr. Peter Green, the tTG enzyme in the brain is in a form called *tTG6*. The tTGs are a family of enzymes found throughout the body. The form in the gut is tTG2, the form in the skin is tTG3, and the form in the nervous system is tTG6. These various forms have allowed researchers to understand the components of CD.

Other neurological researchers claim that the following symptoms are found in fifty-one percent of CD patients, compared with nineteen percent in the non-CD population:

Attention-deficit/hyperactivity disorder
Cerebellar ataxia (disturbances of walking balance)
Developmental delays (slowness in children's speech and coordination)
Headaches
Learning disorders
Depression

It should be noted that any of these symptoms should not be brushed off as CD. Each must be evaluated by a professional.

Research has shown that when an individual family member is diagnosed with CD, there is a twenty percent chance that that person's first-degree relatives (siblings, parents, children) have it also.

The following are some of the complications of CD that have been identified thus far:

Dental enamel hyperplasia. The dentist will see obvious darkening and thinning of the enamel. This could be caused by a lack of absorption of calcium through the small intestine.

Osteopenia and osteoporosis. These are both conditions which show the bones to be more porous and at risk to fracture.

They are the result of a lack of calcium and many times can be reversed by intense calcium therapy.

Anemia, due to malabsorption of iron in the small intestine.

Malnutrition, due to not the body not absorbing most of the food ingested.

Short stature. Many pediatric patients will show a short stature and will start growth spurts after going on a gluten-free diet. At this point, the body is beginning to absorb the nutrients that are so necessary for normal growth.

Infertility. There are many couples who have been treated for infertility and found that one of them had CD. After going on a gluten-free diet, they were able to conceive.

According to Hadjivassiliou et al. in the March 2010 issue of *The Lancet Neurology*,

> *Gluten sensitivity is a systemic autoimmune disease with diverse manifestations. This disorder is characterized by abnormal immunological responsiveness to ingested gluten in genetically susceptible individuals. Coeliac disease, or gluten-sensitive enteropathy, is only one aspect of a range of possible manifestations of gluten sensitivity. Although neurological manifestations in patients with established coeliac disease have been reported since 1966, it was not until 30 years later that, in some individuals, gluten sensitivity was shown to manifest solely with neurological dysfunction. Furthermore, the concept of extraintestinal presentations without enteropathy has only recently become accepted. In this Personal View, we review the range of neurological manifestations of gluten sensitivity and discuss recent advances in the diagnosis and understanding of the pathophysiological mechanisms underlying neurological dysfunction related to gluten sensitivity. (pp. 318-330)*

One of the conditions that is frequently overlooked is a skin manifestation of CD, a very itchy rash called *dermatitis herpetiformis* (DH). According to the National Digestive Diseases Information Clearinghouse, DH is caused by deposits of IgA in the skin, which triggers further immunological reactions that result in lesion formation. The skin breaks out, usually on the extremities. The condition is very difficult to treat because the cause is the antibodies that the body uses to defend itself against the proteins in the grains (i.e., rye, wheat, and barley). Most of individuals with DH have intestinal damage, and many are not aware of it because they may not have gastrointestinal symptoms. DH is the external manifestation of an abnormal immune response to gluten in which IgA antibodies form against the skin antigen epidermal tTG. It is diagnosed by a biopsy next to the affected skin area. If a skin biopsy and the tTG test are positive, that is considered a definitive diagnosis. If either is negative, it is recommended that the person see a gastroenterologist for an intestinal biopsy. There is a medication (called Dapsone) that helps relieve the symptoms of DH, but a lifetime gluten-free diet is the most effective treatment.

John was a career professional whose position required that he travel extensively. He developed a rash that was very disturbingly itchy. He showed it to his physician, who suggested a prescription for a cream and thought it would go away. When it continued, John went back to his physician and explained that, because he traveled so much, the rash was really difficult to deal with. The physician referred him to a dermatologist who took a biopsy and a blood test and diagnosed him with DH. The dermatologist recommended that John see a registered dietitian for counseling, because he had CD. It was difficult for John to understand how a rash could affect the small intestine. After visiting several times with the dietitian, John realized that he had to eat gluten free for the rest of his life. He had to take some food with him wherever he went and had to make special arrangements for long airplane flights and special meals while entertaining or being entertained. He was glad to know there was a CD support group close by when he was not traveling. It was an adjustment, but John found that after he went gluten free his episodes of DH became much less frequent. Within several months, John observed that the rash was less frequent, and he had learned to stay on a gluten-free diet.

As is evident from John's condition, CD has many venues and has effects on many systems in our bodies, if a gluten-free diet is not followed. If a medication to treat CD is ever found, the news will be all over the media and will bring greater recognition to the disease. Right now, however, education is the primary avenue to bring about change. We must educate patients, families, physicians, researchers, public school teachers, church leaders, and playgroups. The more education people have, the easier it will be to cope with a gluten-free lifestyle in all phases of life.

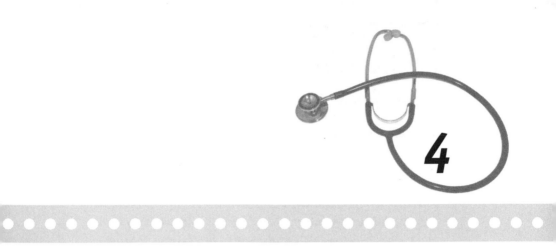

Everything You Wanted to Know About Your Intestines and Other Organs But Were Afraid to Ask

Mother always made me eat a bowl of oats before I went to school, and by the time I got to school my belly was churning. If the oats did not stay down I would run to the bathroom to vomit, but occasionally it would happen in the classroom. Projectile vomiting is very difficult to control. The teacher would send for the janitor to clean it up, and I was sent to the nurse's office to rest until I felt better.

I asked the teacher if I could run to the bathroom when I had to go because I had a hard time holding it in. She gave me permission so when I had a lot of gas or diarrhea I could run out of the room before anyone smelled it. Sometimes the diarrhea was just like water and I could tell exactly what I had eaten. I never discussed any of this with my mother or teacher because it might make them sick.

I was very thin and when I was sent to the nurse's office, she sometimes asked me about my weight. I told her what my mother told people when asked: "I prefer eating vegetables and salads." Now that was actually the truth, because when we had victory gardens during World War II, I would ask permission to sit in the garden and eat lunch. The only thing I needed was the salt to put on the radishes and potatoes.

As I look back at that time, was I eating these items because this is what my taste buds preferred or simply because I didn't vomit, didn't have a belly ache or gas after eating vegetables?

After the school nurse called my mother to school to talk about my weight, my mother took me to the doctor. I was the tallest in the class at five foot, seven inches. My bones were long in length but very small in diameter. Can you imagine being eleven years old, five foot seven, and weighing eighty-five pounds?

When I was in my early fifties, I was working as a social worker for the Texas State Mental Health Department. I went into this field because the doctors had told me that I internalized everything and that is why I had so many physical problems.

A gastroenterologist MD had his office in the adjoining building. I got to know his nurse because we both brought our lunch and ate at the public park adjacent to our offices. The doctor she worked for was from Europe and was doing research trying to find out why there were so few patients with gluten intolerance compared with Europe.

We ate together for almost a year when she asked me if I had ever heard of gluten intolerance or celiac disease. As we got to *know each other she asked questions about my health and I told her how I was raised and that I had been diagnosed as a hypochondriac.*

"You have had all of the classic symptoms of celiac disease," she said. "I talked with my doctor, and he said he would be glad to test you. There would be no charge for the consultation, you just have to pay for the testing." I went for the testing, and it turned out I had celiac disease as my friend suspected. Of course I changed doctors, my health started to dramatically improve and my best friend became my health teacher and supplied me with many books to read and answered my questions. BEATRICE

The body is a magnificent factory that breaks food down to a form in which the nutrients are absorbed to nourish cells and provide energy. This process is called *digestion*. The digestive system is made up of the digestive tract, a series of hollow organs joined in a long, twisting tube that reaches from the mouth to the anus. Other organs also help the body to break down food and absorb nutrients.

Organs that make up the digestive tract include the mouth, esophagus, stomach, small intestine, large intestine (also called the *colon*) rectum, and anus. Inside these hollow organs is a lining called the *mucosa*. In the mouth, stomach, and small intestine, the mucosa contains tiny glands that produce juices to help digest food. The digestive tract also contains a layer of smooth muscle that helps to break down the food and move it along the tract.

Two "solid" digestive organs are the liver and the pancreas. They produce digestive juices that reach the intestine through small tubes called *ducts*. The gallbladder stores the liver's digestive juices until they are needed in the intestine. Parts of the nervous and circulatory systems also play major roles in the digestive system.

Why Is Digestion Important?

When you eat foods—such as bread, meat, and vegetables—they are not in a form that the body can use as nourishment. Food and drink must be changed into smaller molecules of nutrients before they can be absorbed into the blood and carried to cells throughout the body. *Digestion* is the process of breaking down the solid food and beverages into their smallest parts, so the body can use them to build and nourish cells and to provide energy. Good digestion is important for everyone, not just people with celiac disease (CD) or gluten intolerance.

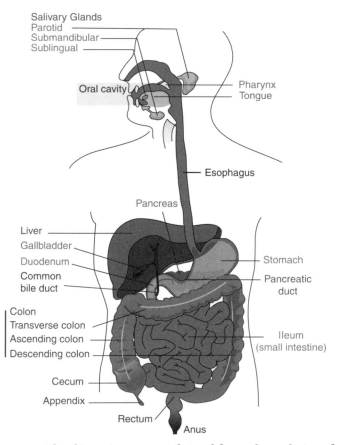

Figure 4.1   The digestive tract. Adapted from the website of the National Institute of Digestive Diseases Clearinghouse, part of the National Institutes of Health.

How Is Food Digested?

Digestion involves mixing food with digestive juices, moving it through the digestive tract, and breaking down large molecules of food into smaller molecules. Digestion begins in the mouth, when you chew and swallow, and is completed in the small intestine.

Movement of Food Through the Digestive System

The large, hollow organs of the digestive tract contain a layer of muscle that enables their walls to move. The movement of organ walls propels the food and liquid through the system and mixes the organ's secretions with the food. Food moves from one organ to the next through muscle action called *peristalsis*. Peristalsis looks like an ocean wave traveling through the muscle. The muscle of the organ contracts to create a narrowing and then propels the narrowed portion slowly down the length of the organ. These waves of narrowing push the food and fluid in front of them through each hollow organ.

The first major muscle movement occurs when food or liquid is swallowed. Although you are able to start swallowing by choice, once the swallow begins, it becomes involuntary and proceeds under the control of the nerves.

What Nurses Know ...

Chew your food well, because good digestion starts in the mouth. Many people believe that if they don't chew enough, then the food will simply take longer to digest in the stomach. Not only is this not true, but also it can lead to problems with your digestive tract. The chewed food particles need to be small enough to pass through your esophagus into your stomach.

What Nurses Know...

Be aware of your food, and try not to overeat. Your body can only break down only so much food at one time. If you eat too much, your body will not digest it until later. Portions of undigested food may even just sit in the digestive tract and contribute to excess, built-up waste in your body—otherwise known as gaining weight.

Swallowed food is pushed into the esophagus, which connects the throat above with the stomach below. At the junction of the esophagus and stomach, there is a ring-like muscle, called the *lower esophageal sphincter*, closing the passage between the two organs. As food approaches the closed sphincter, the sphincter relaxes and allows the food to pass through to the stomach.

The stomach has three mechanical tasks. First, it stores the swallowed food and liquid. To do this, the muscle of the upper part of the stomach relaxes to accept large volumes of swallowed material. The second job is to mix up the food, liquid, and digestive juice produced by the stomach. The lower part of the stomach mixes these materials by its muscle action. The third task of the stomach is to empty its contents slowly into the small intestine.

Several factors affect emptying of the stomach, including the kind of food consumed and the degree of muscle action of the emptying stomach and the small intestine. Carbohydrates, for example, spend the least amount of time in the stomach, whereas protein stays in the stomach longer, and fats stay the longest. As the food dissolves into the juices produced by the pancreas, liver, and intestine, the contents of the intestine are mixed and pushed forward to allow further digestion.

Finally, the digested nutrients are absorbed through the intestinal walls and transported throughout the body. The waste products of this process include undigested parts of the food, known

What Nurses Know...

Mucus protects the inner lining of the stomach so that the stomach does not digest itself.

as *fiber*, and older cells that have been shed from the mucosa. This material is pushed into the colon, where it remains until it is expelled as feces by a bowel movement.

Production of Digestive Juices

The digestive glands in the mouth, called the *salivary glands*, are the first digestive juices within the digestive system to act on the food. *Saliva*, produced by these glands, contains an enzyme that begins digesting the starch from the food into smaller molecules. An *enzyme* is a substance that speeds up chemical reactions in the body.

The next set of digestive glands is located in the stomach lining. They produce stomach acid and an enzyme that digests protein. A thick mucus layer called the *mucosa* helps keep the acidic digestive juice from dissolving the tissue of the stomach itself. In most people, the stomach mucosa is able to resist the digestive juice, although food and other tissues of the body cannot.

After the stomach empties the food and juice mixture into the small intestine, the juices of two other digestive organs mix with the food. One of these organs is the *pancreas*. It produces a juice that contains a wide array of enzymes to break down the carbohydrate, fat, and protein in food. Other enzymes that are active in the process come from glands in the wall of the intestine.

The second organ, the *liver*, produces yet another digestive juice: bile. Bile is stored between meals in the gallbladder. At mealtimes, it is squeezed out of the gallbladder, through the bile ducts, and into the intestine to mix with the fat in food. The bile

What Nurses Know ...

The pancreas secretes enzymes that help break down the carbohydrates, proteins, and fats that we eat. The pancreas is an integral part of the digestive system that often goes unnoticed until problems occur.

acids dissolve fat into the watery contents of the intestine, much like detergents that dissolve grease from a frying pan. After fat is dissolved, it is digested by enzymes from the pancreas and the lining of the intestine.

Absorption and Transport of Nutrients

Most digested molecules of food, as well as water and minerals, are absorbed through the small intestine. The mucosa of the small intestine contains many folds that are covered with tiny fingerlike projections called *villi*. In turn, the villi are covered with microscopic projections called *microvilli*. These structures create a vast surface area through which nutrients can be absorbed. Specialized cells allow absorbed materials to cross the mucosa into the blood, where they are carried off in the bloodstream to other parts of the body for storage or further chemical change. This part of the process varies with different types of nutrients. It is at this junction that it is important to realize the fact that CD destroys the villi and microvilli. This vast surface is no longer able to absorb nutrients from food and can result in malnutrition and many other systemic deficiencies.

Carbohydrates

It has been recommended that forty-five to sixty-five percent of total daily calories be from carbohydrates. Foods rich in

What Nurses Know...

The liver weighs as much as three soccer balls.

carbohydrates include gluten-free bread, potatoes, dried peas and beans, rice, gluten-free pasta, fruits, and vegetables. Many of these foods contain both starch and fiber. Rice flours used in gluten-free baking are usually not enriched. Some of the newer gluten-free recipes use sorghum flour, amaranth, quinoa, and bean flours, which are richer in nutrients and have more fiber.

The digestible carbohydrates—starch and sugar—are broken into simpler molecules by enzymes in the saliva, in juice produced by the pancreas, and in the lining of the small intestine. Starch is digested in two steps. First, an enzyme in the saliva and pancreatic juice breaks the starch into molecules called *maltose.* Then an enzyme in the lining of the small intestine splits the maltose into glucose molecules that can be absorbed into the blood. Glucose is carried through the bloodstream to the liver, where it is stored or used to provide energy for the body.

Sugars are digested in one step. An enzyme in the lining of the small intestine digests *sucrose,* also known as *table sugar,* into *glucose* and *fructose,* which are absorbed through the intestine into the blood. Milk contains another type of sugar, called *lactose,* which is changed into absorbable molecules by another enzyme in the intestinal lining.

Fiber is undigested and moves through the digestive tract without being broken down by enzymes. Many foods contain both soluble and insoluble fiber. Soluble fiber dissolves easily in water and takes on a soft, gel-like texture in the intestines. Insoluble fiber, on the other hand, passes essentially unchanged through the intestines.

What Nurses Know ...

If the small intestine were stretched out flat it would be the size of a football field. It is about twenty feet long.

Protein

Foods such as meat, eggs, and beans consist of giant molecules of protein that must be digested by enzymes before they can be used to build and repair the body tissues. An enzyme in the juice of the stomach starts the digestion of swallowed protein. Then, in the small intestine, several enzymes from the pancreatic juice and the lining of the intestine complete the breakdown of huge protein molecules into small molecules called *amino acids*. These small molecules can be absorbed through the small intestine into the blood and then be carried to all parts of the body to build the walls and other parts of cells.

Fats

Fat molecules are a rich source of energy for the body. The first step in digestion of fat, such as butter, is to dissolve it into the watery content of the intestine. The bile acids produced by the liver dissolve fat into tiny droplets and allow pancreatic and intestinal enzymes to break the large fat molecules into smaller ones. Some of these small molecules are fatty acids and cholesterol. The bile acids combine with the fatty acids and cholesterol and help these molecules move into the cells of the mucosa. In these cells the small molecules are formed back into large ones, most of which pass into small vessels called *lymphatics* near the intestine. These lymphatics carry the reformed fat to the veins of the chest, and the blood carries the fat to storage depots in different parts of the body.

Vitamins

Another vital part of food that is absorbed through the small intestine are vitamins. The fluid in which vitamins can be dissolved classifies the two types of vitamin: (a) water-soluble vitamins (all the B vitamins and vitamin C) and (b) fat-soluble vitamins (vitamins A, D, E, and K). Fat-soluble vitamins are stored in the liver and fatty tissue of the body, whereas water-soluble vitamins are not easily stored; excess amounts are flushed out in the urine.

Water and Salt

Most of the material absorbed through the small intestine is water in which salt is dissolved. The salt and water come from the food and liquid you swallow and the juices secreted by the many digestive glands.

Hormone Regulators Control Digestion

The major hormones that control the functions of the digestive system are produced and released by cells in the mucosa of the stomach and small intestine. These hormones are released into the blood of the digestive tract; travel back to the heart and through the arteries; and return to the digestive system, where they stimulate digestive juices and cause organ movement.

The main hormones that control digestion are gastrin, secretin, and cholecystokinin:

- **Gastrin** causes the stomach to produce an acid for dissolving and digesting some foods. Gastrin is also necessary for normal cell growth in the lining of the stomach, small intestine, and colon.
- **Secretin** causes the pancreas to send out a digestive juice that is rich in bicarbonate. The bicarbonate helps neutralize the acidic stomach contents as they enter the small intestine. Secretin also stimulates the stomach to produce *pepsin*, an enzyme that digests protein, and stimulates the liver to produce bile.
- **Cholecystokinin** causes the pancreas to produce the enzymes of pancreatic juice and causes the gallbladder to empty. It also promotes normal cell growth of the pancreas.

Two additional hormones in the digestive system regulate appetite:

- **Ghrelin** is produced in the stomach and upper intestine in the absence of food in the digestive system and stimulates appetite.
- **Peptide YY** is produced in the digestive tract in response to a meal in the system and inhibits appetite.

Both of these hormones work on the brain to help regulate the intake of food for energy.

Nerve Regulators

Two types of nerves help control the action of the digestive system.

The first type, *extrinsic*, or outside, nerves come to the digestive organs from the brain or the spinal cord. They release two chemicals, called *acetylcholine* and *adrenaline.* Acetylcholine causes the muscle layer of the digestive organs to squeeze with more force and increase the "push" of food and juice through the digestive tract. It also causes the stomach and pancreas to produce more digestive juice. Adrenaline has the opposite effect. It relaxes the muscle of the stomach and intestine and decreases the flow of blood to these organs, slowing or stopping digestion.

The second kind of nerves are *intrinsic*, or inside nerves, and they make up a very dense network embedded in the walls of the esophagus, stomach, small intestine, and colon. The intrinsic nerves are triggered to act when the walls of the hollow organs are stretched by food. They release many different substances that speed up or delay the movement of food and the production of juices by the digestive organs.

Together, nerves, hormones, blood, and the organs of the digestive system conduct the complex tasks of digesting and absorbing nutrients from the foods and liquids you consume each day.

It is very evident that if the lining of the small intestine is inflamed and the villi destroyed, villi would then be unable to absorb water and nutrients such as vitamins, folic acid, iron, and calcium. This causes a person living with CD to be susceptible to a variety of other conditions related to poor nutrition and malabsorption of nutrients.

We are carefully and wonderfully made for our bodies to function in all of the ways described in this chapter and thus far only the gastrointestinal function has been described. In order for the intestinal organs to function, they have to coordinate with the other parts of our body, such as the skeletal, neuromuscular, circulatory, and integumentary (skin, hair, nails, etc.) systems as well as the unseen systems, including the immune, nervous, respiratory, endocrine, urinary systems; cerebral functions; and cell reproduction, which also play an integral part of our body functions. According to Job 37:14, "Listen to this, O Job; Stand still and consider the wondrous works of God."

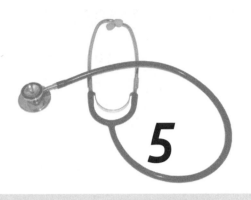

What Is Gluten, and
Why Can't I Eat It?

This seems like the right time and place to say something I've been thinking about for awhile as I'm visiting restaurants. Please encourage people to continue to tell the wait staff, chef, and others that you are a celiac and educate them in the same way you did years ago when no one knew what gluten free was. Why? Because everyone seems to have a different idea about our needs, largely as a result of sooo many people eating gluten free as part of the latest fad or diet to lose weight. We need to reassemble the troops and march on, instructing and dispelling myths aimed at our guts. If they tell you they know all about it, ask them to describe their process. Chances are they need to be re-educated. I've been faced with wait staff "trained" by other patrons who eat gluten free only part time, based on some individual requirement such as how they feel that day. This is maddening and scary! Remember; we have dire consequences if fed any gluten—ever. We need to politely make our voices heard.   JILL

There is no "magic pill" to treat celiac disease (CD) so far. If a pill could cure the symptoms of CD and/or gluten intolerance, everyone would know about it, because it would be on television every day. The pharmaceutical company with the patent for such a pill would definitely advertise, because only five percent of people with CD and/or gluten intolerance have been diagnosed. The company would try to educate everyone in the United States and worldwide about the symptoms, because there would be a lot of money to be made.

Sue, a friend of mine, recently stopped by and wanted to know what I was doing.

"I'm writing about gluten," I said.

"What is gluten?" she asked.

"People with celiac disease or gluten intolerance cannot eat wheat, barley, or rye, because the body thinks they are a foreign substances and the small intestine basically shuts down and will not absorb the nutrients in the food. It is hard to diagnose, because symptoms vary in different people," I answered.

"You've told me about celiac disease, but what does gluten have to do with it?" She asked.

I told her that "Gluten is the sticky elastic substance in bread dough. It is a protein identified as gliadin or glutanin. It comes from the Latin word meaning *glue*. The proteins in the grains of wheat, barley, and rye are very large, and when an individual is predisposed to the genetic factors, these proteins go through the small intestine and cause the body to create antibodies, which produce an inflammatory condition. This is known as celiac disease, but when the proteins go through the small intestine and create symptoms without the inflammation, it is considered to be gluten intolerance/gluten sensitivity and sometimes an allergy."

"OK, I've got it," she said. "When I was a Girl Scout my mother was the leader, and whenever we needed glue, she used to mix flour and water, and it worked real good. Now I know what gluten is. Next time I come over, I'll call first. You told me more than I need to know. Have a good day." She walked out the door.

What challenges we face as we try to educate the public. Even one of your best friends may not take the time to learn about a gluten-free diet. Sue definitely had the time, because she stopped to talk, but she didn't want to hear what I had to say.

Now let's get back to the topic of gluten. Gluten is found in all grains, but whereas the *prolamins* (a plant storage protein) in rice and corn gluten are safe for celiac patients, the prolamins in wheat (called *gliadin*), barley (called *hordein*), and rye (called *secalin*) are not.

Oats have frequently been excluded in the gluten-free diet, and this would make one think that oats contain the bad type of gluten, but they do not. However, oats from all of the major companies have been tested for gluten by major laboratories, and gluten is always present. If a wheat field is planted close to the field of oats, the wheat will contaminate the oats. Wheat will also contaminate oats if the two grains are processed in the same building without taking the proper precautions.

It is all right to eat oats when on a gluten-free diet, but the oats' container must read "gluten free." There are several companies that grow their oats away from wheat and process them in a gluten-free facility. It is worth the time and money to go out of your way to make sure you are purchasing gluten-free oats. If they cannot be found in your grocery store, try a health food store.

What Nurses Know . . .

Always read every label when shopping for gluten-free food. Food manufacturers change ingredients all the time. They are not required to inform customers of these changes.

Meat

The category of gluten-free meat covers all meat that has not been processed in any way. Gluten-free meat has no additives whatsoever or is labeled "gluten free."

Meat that has not been processed and has no additives is permitted on a gluten-free diet. Any meat packaged in a marinating sauce is off limits unless you have read the meat container's label and verified that the meat and sauce are both gluten free.

Cornstarch gravy is allowed, but make sure the seasoning does not include gluten. Many families stuff their turkeys or chickens with bread dressing, and of course we know that is not allowed, because the dressing contaminates the turkey. Cornbread dressing is fine, but again check the recipe and the seasonings used: cornbread, onion, eggs, sage, salt, and pepper make a good dressing.

While at a very large meat market, where my husband and I purchase our weekly meat supply, I asked the butcher whether any of their cold cuts were gluten free. There must have been over one hundred different cold cuts in the display cases. The butcher said she was not sure but that she would check and have an answer next Saturday. The following Saturday she said she had read each casing label and that there was only one gluten-containing product: the honey ham. After all the trouble she had gone to, of course on that first visit we had purchased a pound of honey ham. Then we headed for the health food store, where we purchased a loaf of gluten-free bread. That was a very special treat.

Vegetables

The following vegetables are allowed on a gluten-free diet:

Asparagus	Broccoli	Carrots
Beets	Brussel sprouts	Cauliflower
Bok choy	Cabbage	Celery

Collard greens	Kale	Spinach
Corn	Lima beans	Squash
Cucumbers	Navy beans	Sweet potatoes
Eggplant	Peas	Turnips
Garbanzo beans	Radishes	White potatoes
Green peppers	Rutabagas	

All squash, including spaghetti squash, which can be used instead of pasta.

When learning to eat gluten free, you will realize that there are many foods that require no preparation. It is strange how important vegetables can be to a person on a gluten-free diet. Because grains are limited on this diet, vegetables can fill the roughage requirements that grain once held. In the next few paragraphs I offer some suggestions regarding how to eat more vegetables with a minimum of effort.

Eating vegetables is extremely important for an individual going on a gluten-free diet. One's health has already been compromised, because whether CD, gluten intolerance, or allergies is the problem, the diet likely was limited while the symptoms raged.

Try making a vegetable or tuna fish salad and use a large lettuce leaf as a wrap. A corn tortilla can be used as a wrap, but be sure to soften it in a warm skillet, or wrap it in a clean dish towel and warm for thirty seconds in a microwave. A crisp tostado shell can hold a shredded salad mix but is even better if refried beans are spread on the shell to hold onto the salad mixture; you can top the salad mixture off with some shredded cheese.

Most vegetables can be eaten raw; however, if there is a vegetable that irritates your taste buds, use your favorite dip generously to camouflage the taste.

Fresh vegetables are the best for you, because of the fiber. Try spinach. Open a can and drain the water off. Eat it cold with a little lemon juice. Don't worry about cooking spinach, because fresh spinach is good fresh and uncooked in salads. Canned asparagus tips are very tender and also can be eaten cold.

To guarantee lettuce is always crisp and clean, wash it, pat it dry, and then lay paper towels the length of a table. Lay the lettuce leaves on the paper towels. Roll the paper towels so the leaves are not touching, place them in a plastic bag. Lettuce lasts much longer and stays crisp longer this way.

Fresh Fruits

In addition to vegetables, many types of fresh fruit are also allowed on a gluten-free diet:

Apples	Melons
Bananas	Oranges
Blackberries	Pineapples
Blueberries	Raspberries
Kiwis	Strawberries
Mangoes	

Large frozen bags of blueberries and strawberries can be purchased in most supermarkets. Blueberries and strawberries are extremely good for individuals with autoimmune disorders. A couple of tablespoons over breakfast cereal or mixed with yogurt can be a delicious treat. Peel bananas and place them in a plastic bag in the freezer. They can be used for a breakfast smoothie fixed in a blender. Frozen blueberries and strawberries also can be used in smoothies. I broke my blender with too many frozen strawberries, so I would recommend thawing them first. A filling breakfast can consist of a scoop of soy protein powder, a scoop of ground flax seed, fruit, yogurt, ice cubes, and soy milk mixed in the blender. This combination is extremely nourishing and will usually hold one over until lunch or beyond.

To make sure every person in the family gets their share of fruit, I started serving fresh fruit at the table with every meal. For example, peel oranges and separate into sections and place them on the table with the meal. Apples can be cut in eighths and the seeds removed. Having raised a family, it is hard to see children take a piece of fruit and eat only half. The fruit would be more likely to be completely consumed if it were served at a meal. I have never had fresh fruit leftovers.

Dairy

Unless an individual is identified as lactose or casein intolerant, all items in the following list of dairy products should be part of the daily diet:

Butter	Milk
Cream	Margarine
Cottage cheese	Yogurt

Cheese: cheddar, Swiss, colby, parmesan, Monterey Jack, etc.
Eggs Roquefort cheese made in the United States

Note that French Roquefort (blue) cheese is not allowed on a gluten-free diet. In the process of making this cheese, bread is added and used as a culture medium to promote mold in the French cheese. Roquefort cheese made in the United States does not use bread as a culture and so therefore is gluten free.

Lactose Intolerance

Thirty to sixty percent of adults diagnosed with CD also have lactose intolerance. Lactase, the enzyme that helps digest milk products, is found on the ends of the villi. If those villi ends are damaged, then the lactose goes through the intestine and is digested by the normal bacterial that reside there. These bacteria can cause gas and pain and attract water to the intestine, causing diarrhea. Children are not usually lactose intolerant when diagnosed with CD. Once the adult intestine heals, then lactose can be reintroduced into the diet. Most adults who are lactose intolerant can tolerate hard yellow cheese (e.g., sharp or mild cheddar) and lactose-free milk. Others can use soy milk or almond milk as a substitute. The symptoms of lactose intolerance include diarrhea, bloating, abdominal pain, gas, and nausea.

The best treatment for lactose intolerance is to stop ingestion of all milk and milk products. There are many alternatives, and some milk is produced with the enzyme lactase added. After the symptoms subside, introduce small amounts of dairy by starting with yellow cheese and yogurt.

The following grains are gluten free:

Amaranth	Montina
Arrowroot	Northern beans
Bean flours	Nuts
Black-eyed peas	Pinto beans
Buckwheat	Potato flour and starch
Corn	Quinoa
Flax	Rice
Indian rice grass	Sorghum
Legumes	Soy
Lentils	Tapioca
Lima beans	Teff
Mesquite	Wild rice
Millet	

Many of these grains and starches become contaminated during the milling and manufacturing process. It is important to purchase them from manufacturers who take precautions to eliminate cross-contamination. All food labels should be read carefully to determine the actual contents. If there are any questions regarding ingredients, then call the manufacturer to verify that the item is gluten free. Many manufacturers want the lot number of a specific item so they can verify the process number they used to produce it.

The following grains should be avoided on a gluten-free diet:

Barley	Einkorn	Malt vinegar
Bulgur	Farina	Malt, malt
Couscous	Farro	flavoring
Cracked wheat	Graham	Matzo, matzo
Durham	Kamut	meal

Oats (unless	Seitan	Wheat
verified	Semolina	Wheat germ
gluten-free)	Spelt	Wheat starch
Orzo	Triticale	

Oats are not in the family of wheat, barley, and rye; however, they have been tested all over the United States and have found to be contaminated by being grown close to wheat. There are gluten free oats that are available, that have been tested to be gluten free, because they are grown away from the other grains and milled separately, are available. Purchase only oats with "gluten free" stamped on the packaging.

Cereals should always be checked for gluten-free status. Many are put on the same conveyor belt as used for wheat and other products. As you can see, these cereals would be contaminated. Call the manufacturer if you are in doubt.

Some CD organizations still maintain that vinegar is not gluten free. Scientists have tested vinegar over and over and are certain that the proteins in wheat, barley, and rye cannot go through the distillation process. The only exception to this is malt vinegar, because it contains barley.

That also relieves the minds of many people regarding distilled liquors, which are gluten free unless they were made with barley (e.g., beer) or have had something added after being distilled. Gluten-free beers are now available.

Some ingredients to question when reading labels:
Modified food starch (if it is wheat based, the label will say so)
Caramel coloring (this is currently not being made with gluten-containing ingredients)
Flavorings
Dextrin (this is not currently being made with gluten)
Soy sauce (there are some brands that do not contain wheat)
Brown rice syrup (may be made from barley)
Starch in medications (see Chapter 10 for a further discussion of this topic)

Labeling Laws

A labeling law called the Food Allergen Labeling and Consumer Protection Act was passed in 2004. It requires food manufacturers to declare the source of ingredients when they contain one or more of the top eight allergens (milk, eggs, peanuts, tree nuts, fish, crustacean shellfish, soy, and wheat). Barley and rye are not considered members of the eight allergens, but many manufacturers are including them in their labeling changes. This labeling law has helped the gluten-intolerant population tremendously. If there is wheat in any part of a product, it must be on the label.

A healthy gluten-free diet should include a wide variety of foods. For the majority of adults and children, the daily diet should include two to four servings of fruits, three to five servings of vegetables, six to eleven servings of gluten-free grains, and three to four servings from the milk food group. Making wise choices from these food groups will provide the nutrients needed on a gluten-free diet.

Most of the gluten-containing foods are enriched with vitamins and minerals. Some of the gluten-free foods are now being enriched, but many still have no vitamins or minerals added. It is essential to get these nutrients through your food. When going for the follow-up doctor's visit after being diagnosed, it is recommended to have basic specimens of your blood drawn, for two reasons: (a) to determine whether any antibodies show up, to make sure gluten has not crept into your gluten-free diet (it also verifies compliance with a gluten-free diet), and (b) determine whether your levels of iron, vitamin D, vitamin B, and calcium are all within normal limits.

A bone scan also is recommended after diagnosis to determine whether a lack of absorption of calcium has caused osteopenia (evidence from a scan that the bones are showing decreased calcium or osteoporosis).

Fiber is an essential part of the gluten-free diet. There are many ways to increase fiber in one's diet, including consumption of the following products:

Whole-grain gluten-free flours and grains, including buckwheat, quinoa, amaranth, corn meal, garfava, wild rice, and montina

Flax seed, which should be ground into meal, using a coffee grinder if necessary. Most stores carrying flax seed also have ground flax seed.

Beans (kidney beans, garbanzo beans, pinto beans, and lentils, as side dishes or added to salads)

Rice bran or corn bran, which can be added to recipes or used as a topping on salad or yogurt

Brown rice (instead of white rice)

Popcorn

Nuts

Be sure to eat at least five servings of fruits and vegetables per day, including high-fiber ones such as raspberries, raisins, sweet potatoes, cauliflower, carrots, and prunes.

Fiber is very important to individuals on a gluten-free diet. Ground flax seed has a nutty flavor and can be sprinkled on any food to help increase one's fiber intake. Flax seed also can be added to a breakfast smoothie.

Prunes can be placed in a glass jar and hot water poured over them. After the jar has cooled, place it in the refrigerator. Let the prunes sit for a few days, and they will be moist and plump. The taste will be a surprise.

Raisins can be eaten alone as a snack, mixed in with cereal, or soaked in water as just described in the prune idea. An old friend told me she soaked raisins in vodka, and each day she would eat five raisins. She claimed it helped her arthritis.

What Nurses Know...

Popcorn (without the butter and heavy salt) is a good gluten-free fiber-containing food.

Brown rice is more nutritious than white rice and furnishes the body with more roughage. It is also not as fattening as white rice because the body has to work much harder to digest brown rice. The body uses nearly as many calories digesting brown rice as the calories the rice put in the body.

Popcorn is a good source of fiber and is not fattening as long as it is not popped in a lot of oil, and butter is not added to the finished product.

The National Digestive Diseases International Clearinghouse has provided the following recommendations for calcium intake.

Age	Amount of Calcium (in Milligrams)
0-6 months	210
7-12 months	271
1-3 years	500
4-8 years	800
9-18 years	1,300
19-50 years	1,000
51-70+ years	1,200

Maintaining a gluten-free diet requires persistence, commitment, knowledge, and the ability to change your eating habits in order to be healthy. There are many options now available in health food stores, regular grocery stores, and on the Internet. It is my prayer that I will give you enough information to feel comfortable reading labels, going out to eat, and fixing a gluten-free meal at home that makes you proud.

The following narrative provides an example of how one family dealt with making sure everyone understood about the gluten-free diet:

My daughter, Emily, age nine, was diagnosed with celiac disease in July 2009. It's been an interesting year getting used to the gluten-free way of life. Emily is a very smart and self-motivating girl. We have had our fair share of crying spells because of the

frustration of not being able to eat what she wants or what every-
one else is eating. She is now at the point where she makes the
decision to be gluten free because she doesn't like how she feels
when she "cheats." KIM

Here are a few things this family has done to help Emily in the
last year:

She was feeling excluded at school; she said she felt like her
classmates were making fun of her for not being able to eat what
they eat. I'm not sure they were making fun of her, probably just
questioning why should couldn't eat a school lunch or snack, but
regardless, Emily perceived it as picking on her. So, we decided
the best way to handle it was to teach her class about celiac dis-
ease and eating gluten free. Emily did research on the Internet
and put together a presentation for her class with note cards
and a poster. The poster had pictures of food she can eat and
pictures of food she cannot eat with red lines through them. She
explained to her class why she couldn't have certain foods and
what happens when she does. The kids were interested in what
she was telling them and asked many questions. From that point
forward, there were no more crying spells from Emily about her
classmates picking on her.

Emily has two brothers, one older and one younger. Although they
said they understood how difficult it must be for Emily to have
such a restrictive diet (she is also allergic to eggs), I wanted them
to have a first-hand look and feel of how it was for her. So, they
spent four days (two school days and one weekend) being gluten
free. Jack, seven, cried quite a bit because he was not "allowed" to
have his favorite thing in the world: doughnuts. Michael, thirteen,
also struggled but made a very good effort, even when we weren't
with him. The sibling "picking" they did to Emily now has nothing
to do with being gluten free. KIM

My friend Sue returned two days after I started this chapter,
and of course I was still working on this book.

"Hey, anybody home? It's Sue."

"Come on in, Sue. I'm working on my book, but it is time for a break."

"Here's a peace offering," Sue said, as she handed a plate with a towel over it.

"How sweet of you, but why do you call it a peace offering?" I asked.

"I'm not sure why I was so rude, but I know my attitude was bad, and I'm sorry."

"What is this?" I asked, as I peeked under the towel. My heart almost dropped when I saw what looked like little chocolate cookies. She knows I am careful about what I eat, and look what she is giving to me as a peace offering.

"Aren't you going to ask what is inside them?" Sue asked, smiling.

"Okay, I'll play the game: What ingredients did you use to make these cookies?" I asked.

"Why don't you make us a cup of coffee, and then we can enjoy the treats," Sue suggested.

I left her in the living room. "Oh, my, please make those cookies gluten free," I thought to myself.

"Come in the kitchen, Sue," I yelled. "We'll have our coffee and snack at the kitchen table."

"Now can I tell you what I made, and how I made it? I heated chocolate chips until they were almost melted in the microwave, then I added a cup of gluten-free peanut butter to the gluten-free chocolate, and then I added two cups of gluten-free oats. After mixing well, I spooned a teaspoon at a time and waited for it to cool. That is the recipe."

The coffee had just finished brewing, but I put it on the table and gave her a big hug.

"That was so kind of you, Sue."

"I know I have a snappy mouth, but I wanted you to know I do pay attention to what you say. Friends?" she said as she raised her hand to give me a high-five.

We are now aware what gluten is and how it reacts in our bodies. The lifestyle begins when you make the decision to read labels, educate your friends and families, educate restaurant servers, and learn how to make a gluten-free birthday cake for the one you love.

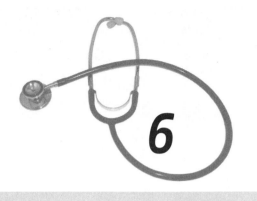

6

How Can I Make This a Lifestyle?

Hi; I am 11 years old and I have Type 1 diabetes, diagnosed at sixteen months of age, and also celiac disease, diagnosed at five years of age. To be gluten free is so much harder than living with diabetes for now. It is a total lifestyle change. With diabetes I can push a button to give myself insulin, but there is not a button to push to be one hundred percent sure that some foods are gluten free. My family has overcome the hardest part of being gluten free, and that is the transformation of a lifestyle.

My biggest challenge is school. I pack my lunch every day, and I cannot participate with some of the school snacks that we have. My mom always makes sure I have a substitute snack in the class so I can eat with everyone else, but you are excluded from the group. Traveling has been OK. My mom researches ahead of time and always makes sure to pack food and snacks. Because I have to be nut and oat free also, we always are prepared. At first we were in awe of everything we had to look for, and my mom broke down in the grocery store because of it. I thought it was too hard to comprehend. I quickly gained control of the situation, and just like diabetes you have to beat the disease and not let it beat you.

The regular grocery stores, six years ago, were not so gluten-free compatible, but because of living on a budget, Mom was able to learn how to cook gluten free using what the stores offered and not visiting a specialty store very often. Nowadays, the regular grocery stores in Ohio are wonderful and have a huge variety of gluten-free items at a reasonable cost. I compiled a list of foods that we have eaten that we did not like so that we did not waste money on them again, then another list with brands of gluten-free products that we like and don't like, quick recipes, and quick meals from the store that we can eat. I always make sure to have a snack available that is free of gluten, nuts, and oats.   DANIELLE

Danielle has a beautiful spirit. She has developed a marvelous attitude in dealing with her living circumstances. Her parents

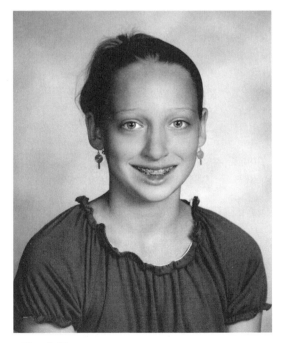

Figure 6.1   Danielle

deserve to take a bow. She is a young lady who lives as a celiac patient and a person with diabetes with grace and courage. I thought you would enjoy her story.

A gluten-free lifestyle is a challenge and a new way of life the moment the decision is made to follow the diet. As with anything in life, there are two choices in decision making: to either *act* or *react*. Acting means each individual makes a conscious decision to do what is best for the body, mind, and soul, while taking loved ones into consideration. Deciding to act requires one to acquire as much knowledge as possible, making it easier to make the right decision. Reacting, on the other hand, is an emotional, childlike behavior, with no thought given to the ramifications to the body, mind, or spirit, or to loved ones. Deciding to act, using one's intellect, is a positive decision, not only for oneself but also for one's family and friends.

> *My mom and dad only make one meal [a day], and it is gluten free for everyone. With work, school, and sports, it is too hard to make different meals. My mom will also make some meals and freeze them. We do adapt recipes to make them gluten free. My mom makes great cookies, pastas, meatloaf, and other foods that are gluten free. She also makes my birthday cake every year that everyone else eats because it is so good. I love to eat out, and we have a variety of restaurants that offer gluten-free items. My mom researched all of them, including menus, and talked to the managers to double check that [the menu items] are gluten free. She now carries a list with her so if we are out of town we still know where we can go. I do not stress about anything. I just go. I am eleven years old, and this is my way of life. I do not stress about anything; I just go with the flow. If you stress about it, the disease is beating you.*   DANIELLE

Living a lifestyle that is different from what you are used to takes time for anyone to adapt. Adults sometime adjust at a slower pace than children, but do not use this as an excuse. We can either choose to act in a manner that makes sense intellectually, and leaves one with a good positive experience, or choose to react to the situation with illogical emotion. The aftermath of the latter sometimes leads to regret and anxiety.

Research indicates there are some living experiences—a job change, divorce, new baby, moving, leaving school, buying a house, death of a family member, or a chronic illness—that are more stressful than others. There are probably many more, similarly stressful situations, but it is evident that all of us have experienced some of these. How life experiences affect a person is up to each individual.

Change is one of the most difficult experiences for humans. Without even realizing it, humans fight change even while knowing it is the best thing for us. This is the reason the right attitude is necessary to adapt to a new lifestyle. Realizing the difference between acting and reacting, and facing the fact that humans resist change, is the beginning of making a smooth transition into a new lifestyle.

If you give it a chance, living a gluten-free lifestyle will become such a part of your life that it is not a burden or a stressor. Read the label—that is a must—and then move on. Do not analyze it to the state of paralysis. We should all be thankful to live in this day and age with all of the knowledge about gluten-free diets. My grandfather died in 1937, at a young age, with a distended abdomen. The doctors did not know what was wrong with him. Then in 1958 the surgeon operated on my father and said "His gut fell apart in my hands; there was absolutely nothing I could do. Peritonitis has already set in." Antibiotics, the ones they had in 1958, did not even touch the infection. At this time, looking back on these situations, it seems evident that my father probably had celiac disease (CD), as did my grandfather.

Gratitude means being thankful for having known those who have passed before us and having shared in their lives. Gratitude for me means being thankful to have lived long enough to know my grandchildren. My father was not as fortunate. Gratitude also is being thankful for now having a diagnosis and a diet to follow that allows us to live a long normal life if we maintain a gluten-free lifestyle. Those with CD who do not follow the diet are not so fortunate.

Spirituality allows you to take one day at a time, knowing that you are doing your best, regardless of those around you. Meditating on a regular basis helps to keep priorities in perspective in one's daily life.

A group of researchers from Italy conducted a study on the emotional aspects of CD in adults. They found that all participants in the evaluation experienced the following sequence of emotions: fear, anger, anxiety, and sadness, followed by reassurance and, last, resignation and relief. Their conclusion was that in adult celiac patients, adaptive and psychological aspects must be taken into account to understand CD and to achieve better clinical management.

Any prior study of the symptoms of grief and loss will indicate that they parallel, as the research just described shows, the emotional aspects of CD. After an individual has lived with symptoms for years, without knowing the cause, it is a relief to know what is happening, even if that person has to eat gluten free for life. The term *hypochondriac* comes to mind, whether self-imposed or from folks who are ignorant of the disease. When you realize that these symptoms have been analyzed by experts in the field, you know that your discomfort is founded on facts.

Each person makes a decision, many times a day, regarding what attitude to display about various circumstances and different people. It is always the individual's total decision as to what attitude to take. Choice was given to each person as a gift. The beginning of humility is the realization that one is able to admit that the only person you can change is yourself. Humility and gratitude are the beginning of serenity, the realization that good comes out of the worst circumstances. If an "attitude of gratitude" umbrellas one's decision to action, with the knowledge that we are unable to change no other human being except ourselves, and a realization of our insignificance in the overall scheme of things, then this is the real beginning of true happiness, peace of mind, and serenity.

All of the ideas discussed thus far can be applied to a gluten-free lifestyle. This pertains to our attitude about our diet and our willingness to always gather new educational resources about a gluten-free lifestyle and to be constantly aware of acting on (instead of reacting to) every situation. If a friend or family member has an incorrect attitude about our gluten-free diet, we can quietly do what we know is right. Our behavior can change another person's attitude if that other person sees our health improve.

I received a note some years ago from a friend who worked as a training specialist at the Lee County Association for Retarded Citizens in Florida. She was amazed at how easily her clients picked up the difference between acting and reacting. She used the following poem, which one of the other training specialists wrote, and her clients recited it as a group.

Nobody can make me happy.
Nobody can make me sad.
Nobody can make me grouchy.
Nobody can make me mad.
I am responsible for what I think,
What I say, and
How I behave.

Mary Bessie, a LARC client, used to throw wild temper fits. She would scream and try to tear her clothes off, and there was nothing anyone could do to help her calm down. The irony of this was that she was fully aware of her actions. She communicated with a few words and some sign language. While getting on a bus one day, she fell and broke her arm. Medics were called to the scene but had difficulty putting her into the ambulance because she was throwing a tantrum. My friend used sign language to her, saying, "You need to act like a grown woman." Mary Bessie was looking directly at her and immediately stopped yelling and said "I'm sorry. I'm sorry." Soon she was completely cooperative going to the hospital and in the emergency room.

If Mary Bessie, with her limitations, was able to comprehend that she had a choice, then people with all the reasoning skills at

What Nurses Know...

About twenty percent of individuals with Down syndrome have CD.

their command should be able to follow through in beginning to develop new patterns of behavior.

It is impossible to change one's behavior overnight, but it is possible to start acting like the person you want to become until you are that person. Try faking it until you make it!

One of the difficulties of a gluten-free diet is the cost. Obtaining gluten-free food is more expensive than buying regular food, and for persons with a limited income it can be a hardship. There are some countries in Europe that actually pay for gluten-free food because CD is a medical condition. (Wouldn't that be nice?)

To begin your gluten-free lifestyle, start with the basics of what contains gluten and what does not (see Chapter 5 for a thorough discussion of gluten-free foods). Make a list of your favorite foods and where to purchase them. If you find a favorite food or mix at a certain store, write it down. Also, it takes awhile, but most recipes can be adapted to be gluten free.

A woman in a gluten-free support group stated that the thing she missed the most was a sandwich that stayed together, so she learned to make sandwich buns to look like they had been purchased at a bakery, topped with sesame seeds, poppy seeds, or onion. They were brown on both sides, and if cut while warm they tasted just like any other bun. This brings a satisfaction that makes one realize that people on a gluten-free diet are not deprived. Delicious buns are now available to purchase at health food stores.

There are so many options available that never existed ten years ago, and more are coming. One of the major cereal companies, General Mills, now offers gluten-free Chex cereals, cake

What Nurses Know...

Be prepared for your first few trips to the grocery store as a gluten-free shopper to be really long. You have to read the label on everything, and you'll have some unpleasant surprises as you discover that gluten lurks in places where you least expect. Take comfort in the fact that companies are producing more and more gluten-free alternatives.

mixes, cookie mixes, and biscuit mix. You can use the biscuit mix for any recipe that uses Bisquick. It is also possible to make your own biscuit mix; just keep it in the refrigerator and use it in any Bisquick recipe. It was reported that a gluten-free Hamburger Helper will soon be on the shelves. It is my hope that by the time this book comes out all supermarkets will have it available. Health food stores usually have a good selection of gluten-free foods; however, still read the labels. Take nothing for granted. Do not be shy about asking the grocery manager to order gluten-free foods. They are usually more than happy to take your order.

Web sites, listed in the Resources section at the end of this book, will assist in ordering food through mail order catalogs. People without a computer can go to the library, get on the Web, and request a company's catalog by mail. The librarians are extremely helpful if one does not know how to use a computer.

Make an effort not to decline any social invitations without giving it some thought. If the event is a formal one, discuss with the hostess what you can and cannot eat. If you are uncomfortable with that, explain that you would love to come but ask her not to be offended if you bring your own food (e.g., sandwich, salad, and dessert) or whatever you are comfortable doing. Or you can offer to bring a dish. Only you will know if your relationship to the individual would make this offer appropriate.

What Nurses Know...

Keep in mind that a lot of fast food is not gluten free. There is also a lot of cross-contamination, and generally the staff are less informed on this option than the staff of a high-end restaurant, so be careful!

When planning a day out, think ahead and plan to take a snack bag in case you are unable to find something to eat. Wendy's chili and baked potato with a Frosty are always safe on the road. (Avoid the french fries, because they are frequently cooked in the same oil as the chicken fingers.) Most of the fast food stores list the nutrition information on their Web site or in a brochure on the premises. Be sure to ask, and read, before ordering.

Remember to always shop on the outside aisles of the grocery store, because that is where the freshest, most healthy food items are stocked. Fresh meats, vegetables, fruits, and dairy products are all gluten free. If a person is also lactose intolerant, soy or almond milk can be substituted; these are found in most grocery stores. Labels on mixes, soups, and canned goods, which are located on the inside aisles, must be read carefully. Many cans or packages will say that the product contains gluten or that it was not processed in a gluten-free environment.

My husband once tried to get me a box of chocolate-covered cherries for Valentines Day. When he inquired at the candy store they informed him that they always use wheat flour on their conveyor belt to keep the chocolate from sticking. He went to three places, and they all told him the same thing. He bought me flowers instead.

Anyone on a gluten-free diet remembers the first time he or she shopped after starting the diet. The reason that it is so memorable is because it was an overwhelming two to three hours. Always allow enough time, without any limitations, to browse

What Nurses Know . . .

The following are some overlooked foods that may contain gluten:

Imitation seafood	Marinades	Processed meats
Sauces and gravy	Broth	Candy
Coating mixes	Meat substitutes	Soy sauce
Thickeners	Imitation bacon	Croutons

through the aisles reading labels. If a few tears are shed because of frustration, please be aware that we have all experienced the same thing. Do not be discouraged because the learning curve is so high. There is enough information out there to help make it easier. Some people find it helpful to make a quick checklist for their family and friends containing their favorite condiments and foods that they enjoy and know are gluten free. The following is an example:

To my family and friends—
These are items that I am allowed to eat on a gluten-free diet:
All meats, fruits, and fresh vegetables not mixed with any grains, Salads without croutons
Hellman's mayonnaise, catsup, vinegar and oil
Spicy mustard
Regular butter, pure whipped cream, margarine (please read label)
Jell-O
Most ice cream (please read label)
Betty Crocker mixes that are labeled "gluten free"
Bob's Red Mill gluten-free mixes
Mixes purchased from a health food store labeled "gluten free"
Please note that many canned products are not from a gluten-free environment, so please read the label.

What Nurses Know . . .

There are over two thousand gluten-free items in most grocery stores, with more to come!

This is just an example of how to handle friends or relatives when invited to their home for a meal. Perhaps it would be better to explain, "I certainly want to attend; however, I am on a gluten-free diet, and I would like to bring a casserole to share. This way I can enjoy the company and I will not go off my diet."

If an invitation is extended to attend a turkey dinner, for example, ask the hostess if she would mind cooking the turkey without stuffing and then offer to bring gluten-free stuffing.

As you may have noticed, achieving a gluten-free lifestyle still depends on one's attitude. Every parent is determined to protect his or her child from harm. As hard as a parent might try, the child will become ill on occasion. Do not play the "guilt game." It is really easy for a child to learn the guilt game and say "Look what you did to me," and never accept the consequences for his or her own behavior. Please do not go there. Education for family and friends will help, but there are still those who think "Just a little bit will not hurt." They are so wrong.

When shopping, always read the labels before putting anything into your basket. All gluten-free products will have "gluten free" marked on the label or will indicate that they contain an allergen, like "Contains wheat." Many food manufacturers are now including the "gluten free" label on regular products. Officials at Kraft have said that they will have a "gluten free" label on all of their products that do not contain wheat.

Be imaginative and try making snacks with gluten-free Chex cereal. There are many recipes on the General Mills Web site that will give you some ideas. They also have contests for using their gluten-free cake mixes and gluten-free Bisquick mix. You may enjoy entering one if you have an exclusive idea.

Smaller local gluten-free bakeries will always be willing to meet your individual needs. A gluten-free birthday cake or cup-cakes for the school class are a few ideas. Everyone from one to ninety likes a birthday cake.

A May 2010 issue of *USA Today* included a sixteen-page supplement on CD, sponsored by vendors of gluten-free products. The most interesting part of this was the positive way it was presented. The supplement highlighted two athletes: (a) golfer Sarah Jane Smith, a 25-year-old from Australia, and (b) A. J. Clemens, Jr., an 18-year-old competitive skier from the United States. These two individuals are not permitting CD to inter-fere with their active lifestyle. As athletes, they embrace their lifestyle and realize how fortunate they are to have this disease in remission by simply eating gluten free. They focus on what they can eat and don't bother to dwell on food that will make them sick.

Children who are gluten intolerant learn to read labels at a very young age. At the annual Celiac Conference at Nationwide Children's Hospital in Columbus, Ohio, there are classes for chil-dren of all ages. Even the youngest learn the necessity of reading labels. The individuals who teach these classes are very creative, even showing the children how to cook gluten free.

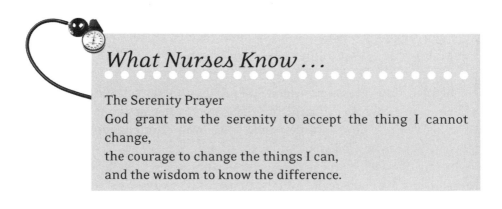

What Nurses Know...

The Serenity Prayer
God grant me the serenity to accept the thing I cannot change,
the courage to change the things I can,
and the wisdom to know the difference.

The American Celiac Disease Alliance's members hail from celiac research centers and celiac and gluten intolerance organizations and include authors and some vendors. This alliance was created to lobby politicians to help advance their goals. They really did a great job when they were successful in getting the Food and Drug Administration (FDA) to add wheat to the allergens list. They have been active in getting the FDA to identify how much gluten is in food that is considered gluten free; they are asking for twenty parts per million, but that has not been decided yet. The FDA's decision on this topic was due in 2006. FDA officials are still working on it.

Insurance companies are still refusing to reimburse their policyholders for dietitian counseling after a person has been diagnosed with gluten intolerance or CD. Because diet is the only criterion for treatment, it is essential that each person diagnosed receive correct gluten-free diet information from a dietitian who is familiar with CD. The dietitians to whom physicians refer their patients usually know about all available resources. They know where to obtain gluten-free food, when and where support groups meet, Web sites for Internet vendors that sell gluten-free food, informative magazines, gluten-intolerant organizations, and conferences, and other information to help bring more comfort to the gluten-free lifestyle. For more information go to the Resources section at the back of the book.

The gluten-free lifestyle becomes more comfortable when you can sit down with little effort and enjoy your food. Pick something new each week as a special treat to tantalize your taste buds. Never decline an invitation, and create ways to celebrate

What Nurses Know ...

Gluten-containing lipstick and shampoo are OK to use unless you plan to eat or drink them. Ugh!

What Nurses Know...

All vinegar (except malt vinegar) is gluten free.

so that your diet is not a challenge but a new experience every day. If a craving arises for a certain treat you once enjoyed, by all means go to the health food store and see if you can find a substitute. With more people being diagnosed each day with gluten intolerance there is much you can do in your community:

Join a support group and get involved.

Help with gluten-free food pantries, for individuals who need a helping hand, or start one if there is not one in your community.

Help raise money for research.

Attend CD or gluten intolerance conferences.

Help send other group members to the conferences.

Start a committee to take baskets of gluten-free food to newly diagnosed individuals.

What a service to the community you can provide! It takes all current folks who are gluten intolerant working together to help newly diagnosed people feel comfortable. All of us working together can educate the public. Remember, wheat content is now on food labels. This took the American Celiac Disease Alliance members working together to accomplish this, and there is still so much more to do.

My daily personal goal is to be healthy. That means staying on a gluten-free diet and not going off of it. Many people will ask "Can I cheat?" Unfortunately, you cannot. There is no such thing as having borderline CD or being "just a little" celiac. You either have CD or you do not. A piece of gluten the size of a grain of rice is considered enough to begin an inflammatory process to damage the intestine and cause the number of T cells to increase. A person diagnosed with CD has a higher risk for several types of cancer; however, the risk is reduced if they adhere to a gluten-free diet.

About ten years ago, a friend told me that her husband had dermatitis herpetiformis. He knew that it was a manifestation of CD, but he refused to eat a gluten-free diet. He ate whatever he wanted for several years. When he became ill, he continued eating gluten. He had three different kinds of cancer before he died. It seemed so unnecessary. Being gluten free reduces the risk of cancer, making the CD patient's odds the same as the rest of the population. A gluten-free diet prevents wheat from stimulating the autoimmune system to make the body susceptible to this condition.

Plan to entertain your guests with gluten-free food. By familiarizing your friends and family with gluten-free food, they will be less likely to be afraid to invite you to their home. There are so many wonderful gluten-free cookbooks that it is possible to prepare almost anything gluten free now. The possibilities for being creative in food preparation are endless.

Begin your lifestyle with fervor and style. Eat gluten free and be yourself, knowing that you are maintaining your body in a healthy manner and therefore enjoying each day, one at a time.

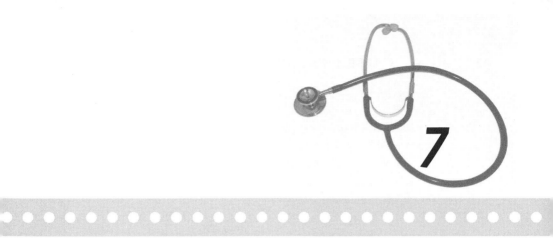

Want to See a Difference? A One-Week Simple Meal Plan

I was used to traveling and was aware that I'm required to stay on a gluten-free diet after being diagnosed with gluten intolerance several years ago. My doctor was concerned about my weight because I was having difficulty maintaining one hundred fifty pounds and I am five foot, eleven inches tall. My laboratory work was showing that I am deficient in several vitamins, calcium, and iron, which indicate that I am not getting sufficient nutrition. He suggested that I go to a dietitian who specializes in a gluten-free diet and discuss my problem with her/him. I checked with insurance, but they did not cover this expense, but since he recommended it, I went for an appointment.

The dietitian asked me before my appointment to keep a diary of all food taken, including during a week of traveling. This really expedited the appointment because she immediately realized that I was only getting twelve hundred calories and I required twice that for my weight, height, and activity level. I was actually starving myself without realizing it because I could not (or did not) eat the right things when I traveled. I did not want to be a burden to my family or my job so I would eat only what I knew to be gluten free and never asked for anything else. The dietitian pointed out that I was depriving my body, and she worked with me for several weeks in developing a plan for a well-balanced gluten-free diet.

I have gained about fifteen pounds and feel better than I have in a long while. My family has been great about my needs, and when I travel I carry foods with me and am now able to ask for a gluten-free meal at any restaurant. AHMED

The American Dietetic Association (ADA) has been very proactive in providing guidelines for a gluten-free diet. Because diet is the only treatment for celiac disease (CD) and gluten intolerance, professionals at the ADA have developed methods for dietitian counseling. They realize that long-term compliance with a gluten-free diet determines the life and health outcomes of an individual with CD. One of the challenges individuals with CD face is consuming enough whole grains that are enriched with adequate vitamins and minerals. If the usual food intake is inadequate, then additional multivitamin and mineral supplements may be necessary.

Prior to starting a gluten-free diet, it is essential to obtain nutritional counseling from a registered dietitian who specializes in this area. Insurance will probably not cover the expense, but the time and money will be worth it. If the dietitian meets with the patient and calls for a care conference, which would include the physician, nurse, specialist physician, pharmacist, and/or social worker, the case could have an optimal outcome, because all parties would agree on treatment and follow-up management of the patient. Some of the factors the dietitian will assess are the results of medical procedures, bone density screening, factors affecting quality of life, gastrointestinal symptoms, and assessment of other disease states (e.g., diabetes, thyroid conditions, and other autoimmune disorders.).

The following menu plan provides examples of ideal, delicious, simple, gluten-free meals. This menu meets the Food and Drug Administration standards and ADA standards, which provide for all daily nutritional requirements, and the gluten-free status is still maintained.

SUNDAY

Breakfast

Four-ounce glass of orange juice
Two scrambled eggs in a corn tortilla with salsa and cheddar cheese
Coffee or tea

Lunch

Mixed green salad with mandarin oranges and raspberry vinaigrette dressing
One baked sweet potato
One broiled pork chop
One-half cup applesauce
Fresh asparagus
One warmed gluten-free banana muffin
Eight-ounce glass of fat-free milk

Snack

One banana

Dinner

Tomato soup
Gluten-free turkey and Swiss cheese sandwich rolled in gluten-free wrap

One-half cup canned peaches
Coffee or tea

MONDAY

Breakfast

One half grapefruit (if not contraindicated for
prescription medication)
Three whole-grain gluten-free pancakes with
tub margarine and light syrup
One poached egg
Coffee or tea

Lunch

One cup gluten-free potato leek soup
Six gluten-free crackers
One cup raspberries
Eight-ounce glass of fat-free milk
(gluten-free soy if you are lactose
intolerant)

Snack

One apple

Dinner

Three-quarter cup coleslaw
Five gluten-free baby back barbeque ribs
Broiled tomatoes with mozzarella cheese, olive oil,
and fresh basil
Three-quarter cup polenta
One whole-grain gluten-free dinner roll
One-half cup strawberries
Coffee or tea

TUESDAY

Breakfast

One cup cantaloupe
Half cup cooked gluten-free oatmeal with one-quarter
cup raisins
and four ounces fat-free milk
Coffee or tea

Lunch

One cup gluten-free lentil soup
One apple
Six whole-grain gluten-free crackers
One carton fat-free yogurt

Snack

One peach

Dinner

Four ounces broiled chicken
Baked potato with margarine
One cup cooked spinach
One-half cup fat-free ice cream topped with fresh strawberries
Coffee or tea

WEDNESDAY

Breakfast

One-half cup cooked quinoa with four ounces
fat-free milk and six dried apricots
One cup apple juice
Coffee or tea

Lunch

One gluten-free English muffin with pizza sauce,
mozzarella cheese, and pepperoni
Small mixed green salad with Italian dressing

One pear
Four ounces fat-free milk

Snack

One-half cup gluten-free pretzels

Dinner

Five ounces broiled tilapia
One-half cup black beans
Two-thirds cup Waldorf salad
(made with gluten-free mayonnaise)
Eight spears asparagus
One piece toasted gluten-free bread
Coffee or tea

THURSDAY

Breakfast

1 cup honey and nut cereal with six strawberries and
2 tablespoons ground flax, served with four ounces fat-free milk
Four ounces orange juice
Coffee or tea

Lunch

One cup gluten-free lentil soup
Six gluten-free crackers
One-half cup mixed fruit
Six ounces fat-free milk (or gluten-free soy or
almond milk if you are lactose intolerant)

Snack

One banana

Dinner

Mixed green salad with tomatoes, mushrooms, carrots,
and zucchini with raspberry vinaigrette dressing
Four ounces gluten-free pot roast with potatoes and carrots

One cup broccoli
One gluten-free dinner roll
Coffee or tea

FRIDAY

Breakfast

Two pieces gluten-free French toast served with
tub margarine and honey
One-half cup blueberries with four ounces fat-free milk
Coffee or tea

Lunch

One cup white bean chili
One piece honey ham and one slice of tomato wrapped in
lettuce with fat-free mayonnaise or Dijon mustard
One cup blueberries
Four ounces fat-free milk

Snack

Four ounces fruit in natural juices

Dinner

Crab meat cocktail (not artificial crab) with seafood sauce
Four ounces baked salmon with olive oil, dill, and lemon
One cup brown rice
One cup sugar snap peas
Gluten-free focaccia bread (a four-inch square)
One-half cup tapioca pudding
Coffee or tea

SATURDAY

Breakfast

Four ounces poached mackerel
Two scrambled eggs

One piece gluten-free toast with tub margarine
and sugar-free jelly
Wedge of cantaloupe
Coffee or tea

Lunch

One-half cup gluten-free chicken with rice soup
Six gluten-free crackers
One banana
Four ounces fat-free milk

Snack

Small bunch of grapes

Dinner

Six ounces red wine
Mixed green salad with light ranch dressing
Four ounces gluten-free prime rib
Baked potato with low-fat sour cream
One cup broccoli, carrots, and cauliflower
One gluten-free dinner roll with tub margarine
Coffee or tea

Meal planning and daily menus vary according to the individual's ethnic and cultural background. You should choose to write out your own meal plan, but these will give you some ideas. Planning also will assist in regulating your portions. If portions are not watched, you will tend to gain weight, which could be a problem unless you were underweight prior to being diagnosed.

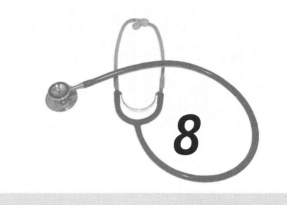

8

Kitchen Readjustments to Make Your Life Easier

As a newly diagnosed celiac, I was very anxious to participate in the gluten-free support group. We were having a conference for about five hundred registrants and providing a gluten-free lunch. I volunteered to come to the commercial hospital kitchen and fix the brownies for dessert. This was a new experience (the kitchen, not the baking), so I guess I was a little nervous. When the first pan came out of the oven, I gasped. They were only about 1/8 inch thick and barely looked like brownies. I realized then that I had measured wrong, but it was too late. They were served as is since there was no way to go back. Yes, I was embarrassed but there was nothing that could be done by then. The lesson to be learned from this is to always read labels and directions, and always keep an unwavering disposition that goes with the flow. JESSICA

The shopping is complete, the groceries have been properly put away, all meals are now gluten free, and the first attempt to bake your own gluten-free rolls is underway. The first time is usually nothing to brag about, but do not be discouraged. Remember that "attitude of gratitude." There is a learning curve for baking gluten free, so you might as well laugh at mistakes and, if palatable, eat them. A mistake might taste better than it looks.

The economics of time and money sometimes dictate the need to conserve resources. Instead of buying gluten-free mixes, try making some meals from scratch. I remember the first Bette Hagman cookbook I received as a gift. She was a pioneer in gluten-free cooking and paved the way for all of us. Her recipes are simple, and her flour mixture is easy to put together. The most recent cookbooks I have added to my collection are Carol Fenster's *1,000 Gluten-Free Recipes* and an Amish gluten-free cookbook from my neighbor Nancy. Besides saving money, a variety of cookbooks give you a flair of creativity and a feeling of accomplishment.

Take a step back and take a good look at your kitchen. Is there a place where gluten-free food can be mixed without contaminating it with other food in the kitchen? Are you planning to have a completely gluten-free kitchen, or are you allocating only a small part of it? Some families go entirely gluten free, whereas others keep a certain section for their special gluten-free area.

Extreme changes in the kitchen warrant a formal 'round-the-table family meeting. An explanation of the problem and all of the possible ramifications of not adhering to a gluten-free diet should be explained in detail. Another meeting can be called to include family members outside the home, and at that meeting your children, if you have children, can help to tell the story. Make sure the children are well versed in the details so they do not have to be corrected when making a statement. Make them a part of the solution and then they will not be part of the problem. Children will not be frightened if they truly understand what is going on. It is extremely important for everyone in the family to be able to get a snack without contaminating the area or food of the person eating a gluten-free diet. They should understand that even a drop of flour or one crumb from toast can make the individual with gluten intolerance or allergies very sick. Take the opportunity, at the family discussions, to place various small crumbs in the middle of the table on a big platter. All should understand how friends can make a mistake when they say, "Just a little will not hurt." A little *will* hurt, possibly for days.

It is mandatory to have two toasters in the kitchen if the person on the gluten-free diet enjoys eating toast: One toaster is for the individual eating gluten free and one is for the rest of the family. The toaster used with regular bread must be cleaned on a regular basis because it accumulates crumbs. If the family has only one toaster, never prepare gluten-free food close to it because of potential cross-contamination. A toaster oven could also be considered instead of a plain toaster because it is more versatile and could be used exclusively for the preparation of gluten-free foods.

It is less expensive to buy different flours and mix them, according to a recipe, than to buy ready-mixed gluten-free flours. However, there are now more ready-mixed gluten-free flours than ever before. A very inexpensive way of buying different flours so you can mix them is to purchase glass jars from a dollar store in which to store the various flours and label the top with a felt-tip pen. To make sure you have the right flour for different recipes, it is recommended that you keep the following on hand:

Bean flour
Brown rice flour
Cornstarch
Potato starch
Rice flour
Sorghum flour
Sweet rice flour
Tapioca starch

Always keep bean flour and brown rice flour close by when you are cooking, because they have more nutrients and fiber than the others. Brown rice flour must always be refrigerated. All of the

What Nurses Know...

Increase your fiber intake by cooking and baking with bean flour and brown rice flour or by adding ground flax seed to cake, cookies, or muffins.

various flours can then be mixed according to the recipes. One jar can be mixed and kept in a convenient place so it can be used for baking, thickening, dredging (meat), and dusting a pan.

There are many variables to take into consideration when arranging a kitchen to safely cook gluten free:

How many people are in the family?

How many in the family must eat a gluten-free diet?

What ages are the children, if any?

Are there one or more cooks in the home?

Are family members permitted to help themselves in the kitchen, to get snacks whenever they want something to eat?

These questions make it very obvious that some kitchen rules must be set in place, especially when children are involved.

There are couples in which one person eats gluten free and the other does not. Many meals are prepared and served, sometimes with a question afterward: "Was that gluten free?" When that happens, just know you did something right. Say "Thank you" and take your bow.

A "safe zone" in the kitchen—an area where only gluten-free foods are prepared—in the kitchen is strongly suggested. If that is not feasible, then prepare the gluten-free food first and then prepare the rest of the food. Cleaning the countertop with a kitchen sanitizer will ensure that it is ready to use for the next meal. Keep a cutting board, not a wooden one, just for gluten-free

What Nurses Know...

All gluten is removed from stainless steel utensils as they are cleaned in a dishwasher.

Wooden spoons and cutting boards are porous and should not be used.

A separate colander is recommended due to cross-contamination.

Have a separate shelf for gluten-free products.

Never use a cooking stone unless it is new and used only for gluten-free foods.

cooking. If a cutting board must be shared, just put it through the dishwasher, because this is the safest way to avoid cross-contamination.

One way for everyone in the family to know what is gluten free, so that no one else will use those foods, is to either use a felt-tip pen or buy stickers. Be sure to mark everything. A mark or a sticker should symbolize that the item can not be double dipped or used with gluten-contaminated utensils. There is now a company that sells stickers for marking gluten-free items in the kitchen. This protects the expensive special items that are gluten free for the individuals who must use them. Stickers for marking items that contain gluten can be labeled "Contaminated." You can also use stickers that are all the same color for to label anything with gluten and use another sticker color for all gluten-free items. This is very helpful with a big family.

Condiments, such as catsup, mayonnaise, and mustard, can be purchased in the upside-down plastic squeeze containers. They are easy to dispense and are not contaminated by someone putting a knife or spoon directly into the jar. Be safe and wipe the opening to make sure a guilty party didn't touch his or her bread when using the product. Peanut butter and butter (or margarine) are the easiest products to contaminate, so they should have a gluten-free sticker or label. There are other ways to handle this problem, but they are risky, so just purchase extra products and mark them "gluten free." Why ask for trouble?

When Georgia was diagnosed with gluten intolerance, she came to my house to try to understand how to set up her kitchen. She asked lots of questions and took lots of notes. She liked the idea of keeping a separate area for gluten-free foods, but she has six children and a husband, and she knew that the learning curve for them might be steep. She and one of her children are required to eat gluten free, so she said that she would fix some things for the whole family and prepare other things separately. I suggested one quick meal: spaghetti with meat sauce. The sauces are usually gluten free (but always read the label), and you just have to add the meat to the sauce, put on two pans of water for the spaghetti (i.e., one for regular spaghetti and one for gluten-free spaghetti) and, while that boils, prepare a tossed salad. I always cook the meat first in the microwave and then add the sauce. Georgia thought that was a good idea and said she was going to try it that evening. She also liked the idea of the stickers, which can be bright red or orange to remind her family that those items are off limits. Georgia was very appreciative to be able to get ideas about how to maintain a gluten-free kitchen. After a cup of tea and a gluten-free scone, she left ready to tackle her new world of a gluten-free lifestyle.

After trial and error, most meals can be adapted to be gluten free. Of course, pizza cannot, but it is possible to purchase gluten-free pizza dough or shells and then make large regular pizzas for the rest of the family. Alternatively, you can make a gluten-free crust yourself, put the toppings on it, and then fix a regular pizza for the rest of the family. That will avoid cross-contamination. So you see, it can be done.

If you want to make your own bread, you should have a very heavy-duty mixer. Gluten-free dough is very thick and sticky and will burn out a light motor very quickly. There are some bread makers that will make gluten-free bread. Before buying one,

What Nurses Know...

Gluten-free bread has to rise only once, so make sure you can program your bread machine.

check with the manufacturer to see if it will handle gluten-free dough. One resource that I have used for that is the 800 number on the label of Red Star Rapid Rise Yeast. The manufacturer's staff are very helpful and have experimented with so many machines and recipes that they can tell you what works.

It is possible to purchase rice flour, sweet rice flour, tapioca starch, and potato starch at Asian food stores. I have done this for several years and have always had a negative test for gluten in my system. Some people feel that these products could have had cross-contamination during processing. The Asian people use little wheat; most of their thickening is done using cornstarch. You must decide for yourself whether you feel safe using these products. As mentioned earlier, there are many flour mixes now that can be used cup for cup in any recipe as a substitute for wheat flour. Those can be obtained at a health food store and occasionally a grocery store. The large grocery stores are now carrying more and more gluten-free foods. I was in a grocery store today and found an unbelievable amount of gluten-free products. I asked for the manager and thanked him for carrying the gluten-free items. You should express the same sentiments to local merchants; they appreciate consumer comments.

You should not purchase prepared foods to bring home unless the establishment is willing to share all of the ingredients used in the product. Many are very happy to do this for you. Even if you are picking up a quick rotisserie chicken, read the label. It is interesting that most of the grocery stores sell them and that some are gluten free and some are not.

What Nurses Know...

READ LABELS – READ LABELS – READ LABELS
It cannot be repeated enough for your own health's sake.

Lactose intolerance is the inability to digest *lactose*, a sugar found in milk and milk products. Lactose intolerance is caused by a deficiency of the enzyme *lactase*, which is produced by the cells lining the small intestine. Lactase breaks down lactose into two simpler forms of sugar called *glucose* and *galactose*, which are then absorbed into the bloodstream. *Lactase deficiency* results from injury to the small intestine that occurs with severe diarrheal illness, celiac disease (CD), Crohn's disease, or chemotherapy. Lactase deficiency can occur at any age.

The February 2010 issue of *Gluten Free Living* contains an interview by Kendall Egan, the magazine's advertising manager, with Chef Richard Coppedge, a graduate of The Culinary Institute of America in Hyde Park, New York. Coppedge is a professor at the institute and has held positions at the Ritz Carlton Hotel Company and Walt Disney World. Egan was invited to observe Coppedge's gluten-free baking course. They started by baking spritz cookies with several different flour blends. They then analyzed the appearance, color, and taste of each kind. Coppedge personally delivered a basket of gluten-free cookies to one gentleman from Montana who had been misdiagnosed for fifty-eight years. It took nine gastroenterologists and twenty-three procedures before medical personnel diagnosed him with CD. He said that Coppedge's book, *Gluten Free Baking With the Culinary Institute of America*, had enabled him to eat again, and he went home with the basket of gluten-free goodies.

When asked about flours, Chef Coppedge said "Weight does not lie. Temperature and humidity do affect all kinds of flour"

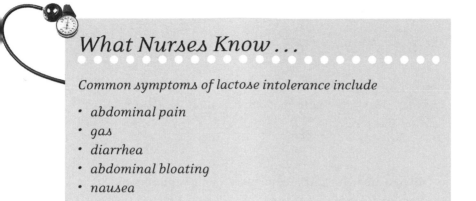

What Nurses Know ...

Common symptoms of lactose intolerance include

- *abdominal pain*
- *gas*
- *diarrhea*
- *abdominal bloating*
- *nausea*

(pp. 28, 29, 44). He recommends that all gluten-free flour be weighed instead of measured:

> *When mixing gluten free flours use only a heavy-duty mixer that can withstand heavy sticky dough. A small lightweight mixer will burn up in no time if it is pushed beyond its capacity. When mixing flours to bake, cover with plastic wrap and use the wire whisk on low and then beat on high. Allow it to settle before removing for storage. (pp. 28, 29, 44)*

These are just a few hints Coppedge offered. His book is extremely informative.

Carol Fenster wrote an article for the February 2010 issue of *Gluten Free Living* titled "Food Safety in the Kitchen." In it, she stressed the importance of cleanliness in the kitchen and especially in preparing gluten-free food. She cautioned readers to watch how you prepare food, watch how you store food, and watch where you put your hands. I will share with you here the top dirtiest things that you touch:

Money
Light switches in public places
Computer keyboards
Cell phones

What Nurses Know...

Do not use a porous stone for regular baking and gluten-free baking. The stone will hold enough gluten to contaminate gluten-free foods.

Toilet seats (which have 295 bacteria per square inch)
Shopping carts
Remote controls
Bathtubs
Kitchen sinks (500,000 bacteria per square inch)
Kitchen sponges

This list gives you an example of how necessary it is to maintain a clean kitchen. Individuals with gluten intolerance have enough difficulty in their intestinal tracts without adding more bacteria. Throw away the sponges and use antibacterial wipes while shopping and at home on all touchables. Fenster suggested getting microfiber dish cloths and using them for only one day.

Food labels are of great importance to a person who is gluten intolerant or has allergies. The Food and Drug Administration (FDA) has standardized food labels, which must have certain characteristics to meet FDA standards.

As an example, Glutino makes gluten-free crackers. They are labeled "gluten free" and "wheat free." The Nutrition Facts on the label indicate that a serving size is eight crackers:

Servings per container 4
Amount per serving
Calories 140   Calories from Fat 45
                           % Daily Value
               (based on a 2,000 calorie/day diet)

Total Fat 5 g   7%

Saturated Fat 2g   11%

   Trans Fat 0 g

Cholesterol 5 mg   2%

Sodium 260 mg   11%

Total Cholesterol 22 g   7%

   Dietary Fiber <1g   2%

   Sugars 1 g

Protein <1g

Below the Nutritional Facts, the ingredients are listed. This is the most important item to closely watch. If there is wheat in the product, it will be listed as an ingredient. Some of the labels will say: "Contains wheat, milk, and soy." Others will just put wheat in the ingredient list. These labels are so helpful, because if you have other food allergies those ingredients will be listed also. Children with CD should be taught to look at labels as soon as they learn to read. They should know what they can have to stay healthy and what ingredients make them sick.

There are some labels that will say, for example, "May contain wheat" or "Packaged in a facility that also processes wheat." If you have any doubt, call the manufacturer and ask of the probability. If potato chips are run on the same conveyor belt as snacks with wheat in them, there is a possibility that the chips are contaminated. Oats do not have the protein that will cause intestinal damage, but a few years ago a company evaluated more than ten samples of oats from the United States and found that almost all of these oats were contaminated with wheat or other gluten proteins. That is enough research to make one realize that you should not eat oats unless they were grown in an area with no wheat nearby. The oats that are sold as gluten free have been grown separately and tested for gluten in parts per million. If they have fewer than twenty parts per million, then they are gluten free. FDA officials have been challenged to identify how many parts per million are allowable in gluten-free food. They have not completed this yet, but when

What Nurses Know...

If you use a long tax form, save all of your receipts, because the amount above your normal grocery bill that you pay for gluten-free food can be deducted.

they do it will be very helpful to all people with gluten intolerance, gluten sensitivity, and CD. So, when you want oats, buy gluten-free oats from the health food store just to be sure they are gluten free.

It is possible to enjoy fresh bread, cookies, cupcakes, muffins, and brownies on a daily basis and, by carefully storing them, to enjoy them for an extended period of time after you bake them. After you bake cookies, muffins, and so on, take them out and permit them to cool. Individually wrap each item and put it into a plastic bag. This goes for bread, too. Cut the bread in slices and wrap each slice. Label and date the bags and freeze them immediately. Then take them out one at a time and enjoy. To defrost an item, microwave it for twenty to thirty seconds, depending on the size. If you refrigerate the frozen items or let them sit out, they will usually taste stale, or crumble, by the next day. Even sandwich buns taste better when frozen and then defrosted right before eating. Toast slightly and enjoy.

Muffin top tins are just the right size to bake sandwich buns. They are about three inches wide, and the buns will become light brown on the bottom and the top. You may use sesame seeds, poppy seeds, or add onion to the dough on top. Slice them when cool and wrap them individually and freeze. You can use any gluten-free bread recipe.

Depending on how many people you are feeding, there are now opportunities to make gluten-free casseroles. Some of the

What Nurses Know . . .

Gluten flour dust can stay airborne up to twenty-four hours after you stop using it.

newer bean and quinoa pastas are delicious, and your family will not recognize that what they are eating is gluten free.

The best news, and the worst news, of gluten-free desserts is that they are usually high in carbohydrates and full of calories. They can be delicious, like a gluten-free chocolate cake, but they can contribute to sudden weight gain due to calories. I found this to be true especially after feeling so ill prior to being diagnosed. When you are hungry the sweets go down easily because they taste so good. This is especially true if you have been ill and now hunger has set in and everything tastes good; this has been my personal experience at least.

We still have to make fruit and vegetable choices and try to add fiber to the diet when possible. A healthy diet will allow the intestine to absorb the nutrition needed, and the whole body will heal. This will increase stamina, clear up depression, and add the vitality everyone likes to experience. No, it does not happen overnight, but as the gut heals and the body renews itself from eating gluten free, we feel renewed and ready to take on the world.

Every attempt has been made to base the information in this book on scientific evidence. It is essential that information be credible and not anecdotal.

The Gluten Intolerance Group has many bulletins on various topics that are thoroughly researched and thus are very helpful to all who are gluten free. They even have documents that can be taken to the hospital so that all of the professionals will have full information on a gluten-free lifestyle. This includes the hospital

What Nurses Know...

Popcorn is an excellent source of fiber.

What Nurses Know...

Check your sources! When you are seeking valid information on CD, gluten intolerance, allergies, or any other health condition, ask yourself: Is the person or Web site providing the information qualified to speak on this subject? Is the information based on scientific evidence?

kitchen staff, to make them completely aware of the necessity of gluten-free food preparation.

Many times, no matter how hard you try, you realize that you are ingesting gluten. If you do not feel well and you do not know why, it could be from something that you are unaware of eating or doing. If you put a lot of effort into living a gluten-free lifestyle, and all of a sudden your health seems to decline, the realization that gluten must be getting into your system finally becomes obvious. Trying to find what is causing the problem isn't always easy. Consider some of the following sources:

- Check the butter container for bread crumbs from wheat bread.
- Check the gluten-free "safe zone" in the kitchen. Has someone been leaving crumbs there?
- Check your utensils. Have you been using wooden stirring spoons or a wooden bread board? Wood can hold gluten.

What Nurses Know...

As is obvious from the preceding list, sometimes it can be difficult to know for sure whether a food contains gluten by simply looking over its label. And there are definitely "hidden" sources of gluten. If you are in doubt, it is best to call the food manufacturer to ensure that you are not getting any hidden gluten in your diet.

- Medicines, both prescription and over the counter, including vitamins, many times contain gluten. Check with your pharmacist. (See Chapter 10 for further information.)
- Fried restaurant foods are sometimes cooked in the same oil as gluten-containing foods. Make sure they are fried in a designated vat.
- Be very careful in restaurants; a restaurant's grilled chicken breast, for example, may be placed in the same spot as a grilled cheese sandwich. Also, many cooks warm the buns directly on the grill when fixing a hamburger.

Alcoholic beverages are distilled, and the proteins of the grains do not go through the distillation process. According to a Gluten Intolerance Group bulletin, all alcohols, except beer, are gluten free. Beer is usually made out of barley, so of course it is not gluten free. There are now beers on the market that are made from sorghum and are available at some grocery and liquor stores and at health food stores, depending on state liquor laws. If you have a recipe that calls for any distilled beverage, it is safe to use because it is gluten free. Also, all vinegar except malt vinegar is gluten free.

There is certainly more to a gluten-free lifestyle than readjusting your kitchen. I am sure that you have noticed many other considerations. It is essential that we protect ourselves from the forbidden grains of wheat, barley, and rye. It is essential that we read labels to know what we are getting from our foods. It is essential that we keep an area in our kitchen that will not be contaminated with gluten. Above all, the most essential thing you must do is to educate your family, teachers, friends, and anyone else who has anything to do with something that you are going to eat. Let's stay healthy by being continuously gluten free.

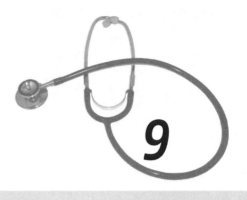

What Happens When I Eat What I Want? Can I Cheat?

I was diagnosed with eczema at age sixteen but now realize that was dermatitis herpetiformis. By age twenty-one I was diagnosed with irritable bowel syndrome, but those symptoms started at age twelve. I had many painful episodes of belly pain over the years and now realize it was celiac [disease; CD] all along. I was diagnosed with Hashimoto's disease, which is an autoimmune hypothyroid condition, in 1994. In 2006, I was diagnosed with low vitamin B12. I went gluten free in October of 2006 after failing a gluten challenge.

I have a hiatal hernia and gastric reflux disease, which they found when I had an endoscopy in October 2007. That is when they did a biopsy and found that I had CD. I was given iron tablets for iron deficiency anemia and found they had gluten in them. All of my antibody tests were positive for CD.

Autoimmune disease goes back at least five generations in my family (and counting), mainly Type 1 diabetes and rheumatoid arthritis. My oldest son has Type 1 diabetes, and my daughter has a skin condition called lichen planus (similar to psoriasis), but she has not been checked for CD (by her choice). When I consider how long it took to be diagnosed and the risks that it puts me and my family at, I do not cheat, nor do I consider it; it isn't worth it. BOB

Sometimes the desire for gluten-containing comfort food overpowers the desire to live a gluten-free lifestyle. Bob's story is a good example of the systemic problems that occur with celiac disease (CD).

If you have been diagnosed with CD, gluten intolerance, or a gluten allergy, then, as you already know the only treatment is totally participating in a gluten-free lifestyle. All three diagnoses receive the same prescription from their health care physician: "Consult with a dietitian, because you must remain on a gluten-free diet for life."

Gluten the size of a piece of rice is enough to do the following:

- Initiate the small intestine inflammation process and destroy villi (a condition called *enteropathy*) in patients with CD and cause those with CD to become predisposed to cancer if a gluten-free diet is not maintained.
- Activate the symptoms of individuals with gluten intolerance, as if a gluten-free diet had never been observed. They may also develop endomysial antibodies without villi destruction.
- Possibly result in anaphylactic shock, actually threatening life without immediate emergency care. There is also the possibility of immunoglobulin E—the antibody that the body creates when there is an allergy—developing.

We may think a person without symptoms is very fortunate; however, that is not the case when it comes to CD. Individuals with CD who have never had symptoms face the biggest diffi-culty. With no observable symptoms, the disease can progress to a point at which even a gluten-free diet will not help. People with CD do not feel pain, and do not experience bloating or diarrhea, but in order to stay healthy they must remain on a gluten-free diet for life. It is hard to understand, without symptoms, that the small intestine is not absorbing nutrients to keep the body healthy.

Some individuals with gluten intolerance complain of foggi-ness in their head after eating gluten. Others will have abdomi-nal pain and/or nausea with possible diarrhea or constipation. The recovery time varies from one to three days. A person with CD causes damage to the small intestine if he or she eats gluten. A person with gluten intolerance will maintain a high antibody count as long as he or she continues eating gluten. Both will def-initely benefit from maintaining a gluten-free lifestyle.

There are many anecdotal kinds of information regarding what to do when you have been exposed to gluten. One of the remedies I have used is to take a psyllium-type laxative (e.g., Metamucil). This seems to push things through the intestine and relieves the pain and other symptoms. Clint from Texas states that club soda really helps him if he accidentally ingests gluten. I have tried it and agree it is an option. There is no scientific evidence, however, proving that either of these home remedies work. The research literature and Web sites have not advocated any recommendations for treatment after the accidental inges-tion of gluten, because everyone reacts differently.

If a person is diagnosed with gluten intolerance and the biopsy does not show any damage to the small intestine, a normal diet could be resumed, but chances are the symptoms will return.

Cheating is a matter of choice. Each individual will make his or her own decision. That is why it is important to have all of the facts when you are diagnosed. If you realize that you have CD and continue to eat gluten, you are at high risk for developing the three kinds of cancer mentioned in Chapter 3 (i.e., T-cell lymphoma, ade-nocarcinoma of the intestine, and esophageal cancer). Continuing to eat gluten when one has CD is a self-destructive decision that has grave consequences. A person who totally understands the possible ramifications of going off a gluten-free diet but intentionally does not follow the diet because of certain moods or attitudes might benefit from talking to a physician about a referral to a mental health professional. If one craves gluten comfort food and foregoes common sense for immediate self-gratification, again, a mental health professional might help.

Once a person diagnosed with CD has improved and is successfully on a gluten-free diet, an annual physical is recommended to determine compliance with the diet. Most physicians will order the following laboratory tests to test for possible deficiencies:

- Total protein
- Vitamin D
- Vitamin E
- Vitamin B12
- Complete blood count (to look for anemia)
- Comprehensive metabolic panel (to determine electrolyte, protein, and calcium levels to verify the status of the kidney and liver)
- C-reactive protein (to evaluate inflammation of the small intestine)
- Erythrocyte sedimentation rate (to evaluate inflammation of the small intestine)
- Celiac panel (includes tissue transglutaminase [tTG], endomysial antibodies, and gliadin antibodies.

If your physician does not order these tests, show him or her this list and request them. It is always good to get verification that a gluten-free lifestyle is enhancing one's health.

The results of these tests will allow the physician and his patient to determine several things:

- *Whether the patient is in compliance with a gluten-free diet.* If the test results are not normal, there may be hidden forms of

What Nurses Know...

Some people with CD have realized they were actually eating gluten—through their multivitamins. If there is any doubt, call the manufacturer of the multivitamin you use.

gluten in the diet that have not been eliminated. Keep in mind that gluten may be found in salad dressing, medication, cough syrup, vitamins, or some other item that being ingested.

- *The amount of healing.* This will verify that the food nutrients are being absorbed.
- *The level of antibodies present.* The antibodies will be normal if a gluten-free diet is being observed. Positive antibodies test results usually indicate gluten's presence.

In rare cases, the intestinal injury will continue despite a strictly gluten-free diet. People with this condition, known as *refractory celiac disease,* have severely damaged intestines that cannot heal, and as a result their intestines are not absorbing enough nutrients. Researchers are evaluating drug treatment for refractory CD, which, although rare, makes the celiac condition much more severe because of the individual's compromised nutritional state.

Rubio-Tapia and Murray (2010) offered the following definition:

> *Refractory celiac disease (RCD) is defined by persistent or recurrent malabsorptive symptoms and villous atrophy (which is destruction of the villi in the small intestine known as enteropathy) despite strict adherence to a gluten-free diet (GFD) for at least six to twelve months in the absence of other causes of non-responsive treated celiac disease and overt malignancy. (pp. 547–557)*

They also stated there are two types of RCD: Type I, which can be classified as a normal intraepithelial lymphocyte phenotype, and Type II, which is defined by the presence of an abnormal (clonal) intraepithelial lymphocyte phenotype. RCD Type I usually improves after treatment with a combination of aggressive nutritional support, adherence to a gluten-free diet, and alternative pharmacological therapies. By contrast, clinical response to alternative therapies in RCD Type II is less certain, and the prognosis is poor.

Paul belongs to a gluten-free support group. He was told many years ago (fifteen to twenty) that he had CD. The symptoms did not bother him to any great extent, so he chose to continue to eat gluten. He lived this way for many years. He traveled for his job and chose not to single himself out for any special needs. Two years ago, he began to have gastrointestinal symptoms, abdominal pain, nausea, occasional diarrhea, fatigue, and some constipation. When visiting his family physician, he described all of the complaints, and the doctor ordered bloodwork for anemia and other deficiencies and the antibody tests for CD. He also referred Paul to a gastroenterologist for an endoscopy. The endoscopy showed that the villi in Paul's small intestine were damaged and inflamed. The biopsy of the small intestine indicated that Paul had Type I RCD. The orders after the procedure were for Paul to revisit a dietitian familiar with a gluten-free diet to ensure that he was following it carefully and who could recommend other nutritional support as needed and for the doctor to determine any medications that would assist in the healing process. Many of the symptoms continued even though Paul was eating gluten free. Close observation by the dietitian and the physician working together gave Paul the support he needed during this time. After several months, his symptoms did subside to an extent, and Paul was then determined to follow a gluten-free diet more stringently and to do closer follow-ups to reduce the risks associated with increased antibodies.

Some areas in China grow wheat, and it is suspected people there have undiagnosed CD. One region where the wheat is grown

What Nurses Know...

Cheating on a gluten-free diet puts the person with CD at risk for many problems, even if that person does not have symptoms.

is Jiangsu Province. Research shows that the genetic haplotypes DQ2 and DQ8 are present in Chinese people, and researchers have encouraged that more studies be conducted to identify individuals with CD. A study of children in China with diarrhea concluded that there are indeed many people with CD, and the researchers recommended that further investigations include diagnosing children.

A study at the University of North Carolina on individuals with proven CD assessed the following three areas: (a) demographic factors and diet status, (b) disease measures (tTG level, weight change, and additional blood studies), and (c) psychosocial status (psychological distress, life stress, abuse history, and coping). The researchers also evaluated number of physician visits, quality of life, and gastrointestinal symptoms. They concluded that, in patients presenting to a CD referral center, psychosocial factors more strongly affect health status and gastrointestinal symptoms than disease measures. This certainly indicates the necessity of support groups and treatment of the underlying depression and anxiety. Several studies worldwide have indicated the necessity of evaluating quality of life issues in the gluten intolerant. The social issues, family situations, entertaining, eating away from home, and educating everyone whom you meet are just a few of the things to consider.

The Canadian government's standards state that no food marked "gluten free" may have any more than twenty parts per million of gluten present in it. This is one of the reasons many Canadian companies, who are stringent about following these standards, market their gluten-free products in the United States. When the U.S. Food and Drug Administration creates a standard for "gluten-free" status, it will be easier for the food producers and certainly much easier for the gluten intolerant.

Dr. Joseph Murray from the Mayo Clinic, the keynote speaker at the June 2010 Gluten Intolerance Group's conference, discussed research indicating that ninety-five percent of children with CD have complete mucosal (healed villi) recovery within two years. Mucosal recovery in adults is less certain. He stated that "One cookie, once a month will continue mucosal damage" and explained that children are diagnosed faster than adults, who tend to be ill and have more classic symptoms.

The Mayo Clinic's Celiac Disease Comprehensive Cascade recommends a complete evaluation of each individual suspected of having CD before a small intestine biopsy is ordered. According to the Summer 2010 issue of *Gluten Intolerance Magazine*, a series of tests, performed as described next, provides the most complete assessment that can be ordered; it can diagnose or rule out CD in most patients. The Mayo Clinic celiac disease center's testing regimen begins with immunoglobin A (IgA) serology and HLA-DQ typing. The genetic typing will provide support for the final diagnosis. An IgA test is performed to evaluate whether the patient is IgA deficient. For patients with IgA within normal range, a tTG IgA test is then performed. However, IgA-deficient

What Nurses Know . . .

A deficiency of the blood protein immunoglobin A (IgA) is the most common immune deficiency disorder. Persons with this disorder have low or absent levels of IgA. If an individual with CD is deficient in IgA, then the tTG test will not be sufficient to diagnose CD. An IgG test must be done, followed by an endoscopy.

patients with CD may not have elevated tTG IgA results. For this reason, when patients are IgA deficient, the evaluation will include assays that detect immunoglobin G (IgG) antibodies. When patients have below-normal IgA levels, both the tTG IgA and tTG IgG tests will be performed. When patients have no detectable IgA, then only the tTG IgG test will be done. This may sound confusing, but the Mayo Clinic physicians are making a standardized approach to CD testing. This cascade approach to testing will allow more than ninety-nine percent of celiacs to be diagnosed.

The National Digestive Diseases Information Clearinghouse describes how different CD symptoms impact each patient. Researchers are studying the reasons CD affects people differently. The length of time a person was breastfed, the age at which a person started eating gluten-containing foods, and the amount of gluten-containing foods one eats are three factors thought to play a role in when and how CD appears. Some studies have shown, for example, that the longer a person was breastfed, the later in life the symptoms of CD appear. Symptoms also vary depending on a person's age and the degree of damage to the small intestine. Many adults have the disease for a decade or more before they are diagnosed. The longer a person goes undiagnosed and untreated, the greater the chance of developing long-term complications.

Researchers have been examining a hopeful new option for looking at the small intestine in which the patient swallows a small capsule, containing a camera, that permits the

What Nurses Know...

An IgG test measures levels of immunoglobulin G (antigliadin antibodies), which are part of our immune system that show whether gliadin (wheat protein) is in the body.

gastroenterologist to watch the video as the camera goes through the intestine. If the villi are destroyed or flattened, this will show up on the video. The only disadvantage to this procedure is that it does not allow for a biopsy.

The Food Allergen Labeling and Consumer Protection Act, which took effect on January 1, 2006, requires food labels to clearly identify wheat and other common food allergens in the product's list of ingredients. It also requires the U.S. Food and Drug Administration to develop and finalize rules for the use of the term "gluten free" on product labels. We are all looking forward to that day.

Jenny is the mother of a ten-year-old girl, Sophie, who has CD. Sophie was diagnosed at age six. She complained of a continuous dull and occasional sharp pain in her abdomen. Her physician gave her medication for reflux, but she had no relief. Sophie's grandmother, a registered nurse, encouraged her daughter to insist on more testing or to change doctors. Jenny was glad she followed her mother's advice, because Sophie was diagnosed with CD. Jenny said her biggest challenge was realizing the responsibility she had to keep her child healthy. She began by educating the family, teachers, and friends. She routinely meets with every one of Sophie's teachers and provides the classrooms with a sealed box of snacks in case there is a celebration, so that Sophie will never feel left out.

Sophie's grandmother loves to bake, and she uses Nearly Normal (brand name) flour and bakes cookies, cakes, and muffins just for Sophie. Sophie has two siblings, ages nine and seven, and neither has CD; however, they are very supportive and know that this is the way that Sophie has to eat.

Jenny has a goal: "CD does not have to define who Sophie is." She has taken the attitude that this disease should not stop Sophie from doing anything.

The family's church is very supportive and offers a gluten-free host for communion. Jenny said that the most important thing that she does is continually educate everyone so they are aware of CD and the effect it has on her child.

The interesting fact is that parents take such a personal, defensive stand when it comes to taking care of their child. They know that in order for the child to get what is necessary, they must educate, intervene when necessary, and teach the child how to live with the disease. Sophie has gone to every Gluten-Free Gang (a CD support group) conference, has attended the group's child conferences, has learned how to read labels and to make choices, and lives life to the fullest.

Even children have to be taught not to cheat on a gluten-free diet. It is a matter of choice to maintain good health or live with pain in an undernourished body. The best way to help your child stay gluten free and not cheat when away from home is by planning snacks and meals ahead of time. Having an honest conversation with your child, when he or she is old enough, may help. And, as always, lead by example: Don't cheat yourself!

Someone with gluten intolerance who has a normal biopsy and does not have an autoimmune condition, but eats gluten, may have symptoms but will not have damage to the villi of the small intestine. The symptoms they have may be uncomfortable but are not life threatening.

What Nurses Know...

Tips for keeping your child or teen on a gluten-free diet:

- *Encourage your child to eat meals at home or pack gluten-free meals to eat at school or on the go.*
- *Work with your child and a nutritionist, and speak to someone at the child's school to find gluten-free foods on the school breakfast and lunch menus.*
- *If you are planning to go out to eat at a restaurant, either choose one that has a gluten-free menu or speak with the restaurant manager to identify gluten-free menu items before ordering.*

On the other hand, an individual with CD who does not stay on a gluten-free diet will experience inflammatory change in the villi, which will eventually be destroyed, permitting the gluten to pass through the wall of the small intestine ("leaky gut") and, regardless of symptoms, start the damaging process and possibly go through all parts of the body. The risk is just not worth it.

A gluten-free diet is the only means of CD treatment, and people who do not stay on such a diet will not absorb the nutrients necessary for a healthy body. The American Dietetic Association has expressed concern regarding a gluten-free diet because gluten-free flours (rice, potato starch, tapioca starch) previously used for preparing baked goods are not enriched (i.e., not fortified with vitamins and minerals). In more recent years, their work has become fruitful as more and more gluten-free bakeries have begun using enriched gluten-free flours. Bean flour, amaranth, sorghum, and quinoa have more nourishment than rice, potato starch, and tapioca flour. It is important to look at the nutritional value of all ingredients to make sure that you get the nutrients that your body requires.

Malnutrition is a disparity between the amount of food and other nutrients that the body needs and the amount that it is receiving. This imbalance is most frequently associated with undernutrition, and in the case of CD it is due to the body not absorbing the necessary nutrients. For example, if the small intestine is inflamed and the villi are destroyed, then deficiencies in the following nutrients could cause health problems:

- *Anemia.* According to the www.womenshealth.gov Web site, anemia occurs when you have fewer than the normal number of red blood cells in your blood, or when the red blood cells in your blood don't have enough *hemoglobin*, a protein that gives the red color to your blood. Its main job is to carry oxygen from your lungs to all parts of your body. If you have anemia, your blood does not carry enough oxygen to all the parts of your body. Without oxygen, your organs and tissues cannot work as well as they should. Anemia in CD is caused by lack of iron due to the inability of the small intestine to absorb it.

- *Vitamin A.* Vitamin A comprises a group of compounds that play an important role in vision, bone growth, reproduction, cell division, and cell differentiation (the process by which a cell becomes part of the brain, muscle, lungs, blood, or other specialized tissue.) Vitamin A helps regulate the immune system, which helps prevent or fight off infections by making white blood cells that destroy harmful bacteria and viruses. Vitamin A also may help lymphocytes (a type of white blood cell) fight infections more effectively.

- *Vitamin D.* Vitamin D is a nutrient found in some foods that is needed for health and to maintain strong bones. It does so by helping the body absorb calcium (one of bone's main building blocks) from food and supplements. People who get too little vitamin D may develop soft, thin, and brittle bones, a condition known as *rickets* in children and *osteomalacia* in adults. Vitamin D is important to the body in many other ways as well. For example, muscles need it to move, nerves need it to carry messages between the brain and every body part, and the immune system needs it to fight off invading bacteria and viruses. Together with calcium, vitamin D also helps protect older adults from osteoporosis. Vitamin D is found in cells throughout the body. The body also absorbs vitamin D from the sun. Some nutrition books recommend that 15 minutes in the sun is adequate for daily vitamin D needs.

- *B Vitamins.* The B vitamins come in many forms.

   Thiamine (vitamin B1) helps the body cells convert carbohydrates into energy. It is also essential for the functioning of the heart, muscles, and nervous system.

   Riboflavin (vitamin B2) also is a type of B vitamin. It is *water soluble*, which means it is not stored in the body; if the body can't use all of the vitamin, the extra leaves the body through the urine. You must replenish the vitamin every day. Riboflavin works with the other B vitamins. It is important for body growth and red blood cell production and helps in releasing energy from carbohydrates.

Niacin (vitamin B3) assists in the functioning of the digestive system, skin, and nerves. It is also important for the conversion of food to energy.

Pantothenic acid (vitamin B5) and *biotin* are both types of B vitamins. Like riboflavin, they are water soluble. Therefore, these vitamins must be replaced every day. Pantothenic acid and biotin are essential to growth. They help the body break down and use food. This is called *metabolism.* Pantothenic acid helps break down carbohydrates, proteins, and fats. Biotin also helps break down proteins and carbohydrates.

Vitamin B6 also is a water-soluble vitamin. It helps the immune system produce the antibodies needed to fight many diseases. Vitamin B6 helps maintain normal nerve function and form red blood cells. The body uses it to help break down proteins. The more protein you eat, the more vitamin B6 you need.

Vitamin B12 is a water-soluble vitamin. Unlike other water-soluble vitamins, however, vitamin B12 is special, because the body can store it for years in the liver. Vitamin B12, like the other B vitamins, is important for metabolism. It helps in the formation of red blood cells and in the maintenance of the central nervous system.

Folate (vitamin B9) occurs naturally in food. The synthetic form of this vitamin is called *folic acid.* Folic acid is well tolerated in amounts found in fortified foods and supplements. It is frequently used in combination with other B vitamins in vitamin B complex formulations.

- *Calcium.* You have more calcium in your body than any other mineral. Calcium has many important jobs. The body stores more than ninety-nine percent of its calcium in the bones and teeth to help make and keep them strong. The rest of the calcium is found throughout the body in blood, muscles, and the fluid between cells. Your body needs calcium to help muscles and blood vessels contract and expand, to secrete hormones and enzymes, and to send messages through the nervous system. It is not uncommon to see osteopenia or osteoporosis in adult celiacs that is due to the lack of calcium absorption in their bones.

● *Fiber* is a substance found in plants. Dietary fiber, the kind you eat, is in fruits, vegetables, and grains. It is the part of the

What Nurses Know...

"Signs That You May Have Celiac Disease," an article written by Diana Kohnle, recently was published by HealthDay News. The following list includes some typical symptoms; however, not every person with CD has noticeable symptoms. Kohnle stated that, according to the National Digestive Diseases Information Clearinghouse, CD may trigger the following warning signs in children:

• *Loss of weight*
• *Pain and bloating in the abdomen*
• *Persistent diarrhea*
• *Vomiting*
• *Constipation*
• *Irritability*
• *Stools that are light in color, fatty, or have a foul odor*

In adults, symptoms are more likely to include

• *Anemia*
• *Fatigue*
• *Bone or joint pain*
• *Osteoporosis*
• *Depression or anxiety*
• *Numbness in the extremities*
• *Missed menstrual periods*

plant that your body can't digest, yet it is an important part of a healthy diet. It adds bulk to your diet and makes you feel full faster, helping you control your weight. Fiber helps digestion and helps prevent constipation. There are two types of fiber: (a) soluble fiber, which dissolves in water and is clear, and (b) insoluble fiber, which will dissolve but becomes gel-like if it sits.

All of the nutrients just listed are needed in our daily diets. Although remaining gluten free is a choice, it is also obvious as to what happens to our bodies if we do not chose to do so.

When you see images of very young children in third world countries with very large abdomens and tiny arms and legs, that is a sign of malnutrition. Your small intestine does most of the digesting of the foods you eat. If you have a malabsorption syndrome, your small intestine cannot absorb nutrients from foods. Untreated CD is a serious malabsorption problem. Fortunately, CD rarely gets to that stage. When it is diagnosed, and if a gluten-free diet is followed, the body recovers from that state of being deprived and begins to heal.

As has been continuously pointed out, the symptoms in CD can be typical or even nonexistent. Silent CD can still produce the inflammatory process without symptoms. I hope that each person who reads this will recognize themselves or a relative and that it precipitates a diagnosis as soon as possible so the road toward healing and a healthy, gluten-free lifestyle can begin.

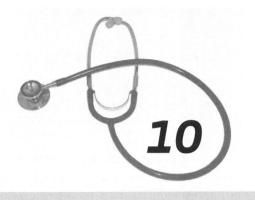

10

Gluten in Medications and Other Pitfalls to Watch For

I attended a conference at Nationwide Children's Hospital in Columbus, Ohio, last fall. It was wonderful to see so many people with the same questions that I have about celiac disease (CD). I have been having symptoms as though I am getting gluten in my diet, but I have been so careful about what I eat and where I eat that I have been unable to determine where it is coming from. One of the speakers at the conference was Steve Plogsted, a pharmacist who has his own Web site, www.gluten-freedrugs.com. He talked about how frequent medications can have gluten in them and ways to determine which are gluten free.

After hearing his talk and being able to ask questions, I determined that two of my medications did contain gluten. It was also in the multivitamin that I take every day. I was so shocked to

realize that was the source but also very relieved to know that I
would soon be feeling better.　NORMA

Living a gluten-free lifestyle means looking for gluten in the most unlikely places. When you look at a pill there is no way to tell whether there is gluten in it. It is wise to have your physician write on every prescription that you require it to be gluten free. If you have a regular pharmacist, you can talk to him or her and ask him or her to make sure that the drugs that you receive are gluten free. Pharmaceutical companies often add inactive ingredients to their products, and one of those ingredients could be gluten.

Pharmacist Steve Plogsted has spent a good bit of time contacting pharmaceutical companies to determine the gluten status of medications:

Excipients are pharmacologically inactive substances that are included in the final formulation of the drug product. Their purpose is multifunctional. They provide bulk to the product, allow for the drug to be dissolved and absorbed at different rates in the body (as in extended release formulations), decrease stomach upset, protect the product from moisture contamination, and simply make the final drug appearance more pleasing to the eye of the consumer. The shape, color and appearance help in the identification of the drug. The [U.S. Food and Drug Administration] has the authority to approve all drug products produced for legal use in the United States. Each drug product must undergo rigorous testing before it can be approved for marketing to the consumer. The proprietary or "brand name" drugs have to meet standards for dissolution, absorption, blood levels, product stability and several other factors. The manufacturing facilities where the drugs are produced must maintain standards in regards to quality control, cleanliness, and packaging. (quoted by Ratner, 2010, p. 58)

What Nurses Know...

The U.S. Food and Drug Administration has the authority to approve all drug products produced for legal use in the United States. It requires the manufacturer (pharmaceutical company) to meet many standards before it approves a drug for distribution. It usually takes over ten years to put a new drug on the market.

Amy Ratner wrote an article for *Gluten-Free Living* about gluten in drugs. She mentioned that the U.S. Food and Drug Administration (FDA), which oversees drug labeling, does not require labels to note when gluten, or even allergens such as wheat, are used. She referred to the Perrigo Company, which is one of the largest manufacturers of store-brand medications. Perrigo is starting to offer products voluntarily labeled "gluten-free" labeling to retailers who request it.

The active ingredient in medications, whether they are prescription or over the counter, is nearly certain to be gluten free. The active ingredient is the part of a pill, capsule, or liquid that actually treats your illness or condition. It makes up a small portion of each dose of medication. Inactive ingredients (*excipients*) make up the bulk of the medication and is where the questionable ingredients could be.

One way to ensure that you will obtain gluten-free drugs is to make friends with your pharmacist. Remind him or her every time you obtain a prescription that it must be gluten free. Many times a physician will write a prescription and the insurance company will insist on a generic form of the drug. You may have to call the insurance company and explain that the brand name is gluten free but the generic is not (or vice versa). I personally wrote a letter to my insurance company telling them why I cannot take pills containing wheat, barley, or rye. I asked my physician to also sign the letter. When I changed insurance companies the old company even forwarded this information to the new one. Call the insurance company to get approval and then write a detailed letter to be part of your files. Do not hesitate to call the insurance company to get what you need. You can ask for a case manager, who is usually a nurse, who is there to help you.

For over-the-counter vitamins, pain relievers, or other medications, carry your cell phone to the store with you so you can call the pharmaceutical company from the store. They will always ask you what the lot number is, and with the medication right there on the shelf you will be able to answer that. The customer service staff are very accommodating and will usually tell you to call each time you purchase a product because the different lots of over-the-counter drugs are manufactured separately.

If you are having any outpatient radiology procedure, call the area where it is to be done and ask the staff to verify with the radiologist that the contrast material is gluten free.

Steve Plogsted spoke at a Gluten Intolerance Group conference and discussed fiber supplements:

> The best way to get your fiber is through fruits and vegetables. When that is not possible, supplements are the next preferred choice. The rule of thumb for adults is 35 grams of fiber per day. A soluble fiber dissolves completely and is clear. An insoluble fiber supplement forms a gel-like solid

What Nurses Know ...

Know the following for every medication that you take:
Name of the medication
Dosage
Reason it was ordered
How often to take it
How long you will be on it

after sitting. This type is better for gut health. For example, Metamucil (psyllium) is most commonly used. The powders are generally gluten free. The tablets or wafers can contain gluten. Medications can stick to the fiber supplement, which reduces the amount of medication getting into the body. Common medications with this concern include all of the following: digoxin, aspirin, Tegretol, lithium, warfarin (Coumadin), fluroquinolones [sic] (Cipro, Levaquin, Avelox), and levothyroxin [sic] (Synthroid).

Be sure to check with the pharmacist before adding anything to your medication regime[n]. (Source and page no.?)

The National Foundation for Celiac Awareness is a nonprofit organization whose Web site (http://www.celiaccentral.org) lists gluten-free medications. It also lists the problems that currently occur because of the lack of controls, which are:

- No current requirements for labeling gluten or allergens in drug ingredients
- No precautions for individuals with CD in labeling
- Lack of recognition among health care professionals regarding potential sources of gluten in medication excipients
- Lack of specificity regarding botanical sources of starch
- Generic formulations that may include different excipients than the brand-name drug.

This list gives a good example of why we must question every medication and the ingredients in it. In cases of prescription drugs, we cannot read the label because the excipients are not listed. If the pharmacist is not aware of exactly what the excipients in a certain drug are, call the drug manufacturer or go to http://www.celiaccentral.org.

Hypothyroidism has been found to be associated with CD. If you take a thyroid supplement, do so on an empty stomach. Thyroid medication regulation requires patience. Keep track of your energy levels. Have your physician check your thyroid two

What Nurses Know...

Starches found in medications:

Corn	Modified starch (source not specified)
Potato	Pregelatinized starch (source not specified)
Wheat	Tapioca

Pregelatinized modified starch (source not specified)

Starch derivatives:
Dextrates (source not specified)
Dextrin (source not specified)

Other excipients:
Dextramaltose (when barley malt is used)
Caramel coloring (when barley malt is used)

times a year and, as with all medications, be proactive and learn what your medication should do when it is working properly, so you can assess the efficacy yourself.

Two other conditions that are frequently associated with CD are depression and anxiety. It is not unusual for newly diagnosed older celiacs to be put on antidepressants such as Zoloft, Paxil, or Prozac. These medications help in controlling the anxiety and feelings of helplessness that occurs in some patients. Sometimes this is just a temporary situation, and other times the patient must continue on the medication. Be sure to communicate with your physician if these problems apply to you and, if necessary, seek counseling. German researchers compared levels of anxiety and depression in adult celiac patients on a gluten-free diet. There were 441 adult patients with CD and 235 age- and sex-matched patients with inflammatory bowel disease. Women with CD were found to have a higher level of anxiety. The researchers recommend that female celiacs on a gluten-free diet be screened for anxiety.

There have been many discussions regarding whether or not individuals with gluten intolerance and/or CD should take multivitamins. Because these conditions are involved with absorption issues and the individual may have malnutrition, it is usually recommended that a multivitamin that includes the B vitamins be taken daily. Foods with the B vitamin complex are generally in grains that are being avoided by celiacs. The B vitamins are water soluble and should be consumed daily.

Obtaining all of our nourishment from wholesome foods is certainly ideal, but in the case of CD the nutrients may need to be replaced until the small intestine heals and the body is showing evidence of good health. Children are good examples: If they have CD, they will not show any growth while they are ill. Once they are gluten free, they start growing again.

Questions still arise about how much gluten will make you sick and what the measurements "twenty parts per million," "ten parts per million," and "five parts per million" really mean. Two support group organizations—the Gluten Intolerance Group (GIG) and the Celiac Sprue Association (CSA)—are proactive in promoting certification programs for gluten-free products. They have set out specific requirements that food makers must meet to use either of the group's symbol on their product.

The GIG was the first national support group to launch a certification program in the United States giving companies permission to use their Gluten-Free Certification Organization (GFCO) symbol after all qualifications have been met. Each product bearing the symbol must have been tested and found to have fewer than ten parts per million of gluten from wheat, barley, or rye. The ingredients must have been reviewed and food processing plants inspected. On its Web site (http://www.gfco.org) GFCO says that it "provides an independent service to supervise gluten-free food production according to consistent, defined, science based standards that are confirmed with field inspections."

The CSA has a seal that assures consumers that a product does not have any wheat, oats, barely, or rye, or any ingredients made from those grains. The CSA still considers oats unsafe for

What Nurses Know . . .

How do you monitor your compliance with a gluten-free diet? The following are some suggestions.

Look closely at your gluten-free dietary pattern.
Ask for at least a yearly antibody level check for the presence of gluten antibodies.
Closely examine all factors of your dietary environment to see whether there has been any cross-contamination.
Look for hidden sources of gluten in foods, medications, and supplements.

individuals on a gluten-free diet. Products with the CSA seal must test to fewer than five parts per million of gluten using the same type of test recently approved by the *Codex Alimentarius*, a document that sets international standards for gluten-free labeling (discussed further later in this chapter).

An article in the March 2009 issue of *Gluten-Free Living* stated that both the GFCO and CSA require foods to meet stricter standards than those proposed for gluten-free foods by the FDA. The FDA is proposing to allow processed ingredients to be considered gluten free if they contain fewer than twenty parts per million of gluten.

The *Codex Alimentarius* (Latin for "food code" or "food book") is a collection of internationally recognized standards, codes of practice, guidelines, and other recommendations relating to foods, food production, and food safety. Its texts are developed and maintained by the Codex Alimentarius Commission, a body that was established in 1963 by the Food and Agriculture Organization of the United Nations and the World Health Organization. The commission's main stated aims are to protect the health of consumers and ensure fair practices in the

What Nurses Know...

Under the proposed FDA definition, products that are labeled "gluten free" cannot contain the following:

- *Wheat, barley, or rye*
- *An ingredient made from wheat, barley, or rye that has not been processed to remove gluten protein*
- *An ingredient made from wheat, barley, or rye that has been processed to remove gluten if the use of the ingredient results in the presence of more that twenty parts per million of gluten in the food*
- *A total of more that twenty parts per million of gluten from all sources, including cross-contamination*

international food trade. The *Codex Alimentarius* is recognized by the World Trade Organization as an international reference point for the resolution of disputes concerning food safety and consumer protection. The reason this information is included here is to make you aware that there is a standardization for world food production. Even the FDA follows these standards.

Jillian Sarno wrote an article for *Gluten Intolerance Group Magazine* titled "When Belly Troubles Don't Subside." In it, she discussed the consequences of CD:

> *It affects virtually all systems of the body. The mechanism through which this happens is the destruction and flattening of the villi. With the absorptive capacity of the small intestine severely compromised, the most powerful consequence of CD is malabsorption: your body cannot absorb nutrients from the food that you eat. Malabsorption is responsible for most of the related conditions and complications of celiac disease, including*

(but not limited to): osteoporosis, anemia, enamel defects, skin conditions and even certain malignancies.

Malabsorptions also weakens digestions further, by worsening overgrowth of "bad" bacteria in the gut and compromising several organs that support and aid in digestion. The stomach, liver and pancreas all produce unique digestive factors including acids, bile and enzymes. When our bodies are not getting proper nutrition to make these products, they become less available. As a result, food is not appropriately broken down, virus[es] and other pathogens are not rendered harmless, and the result is that these large molecules and pathogens are able to pass through the permeable gut border and cause more immune reaction and inflammatory responses. This is how people with CD develop additional food sensitivities and other autoimmune conditions. (pp. 4, 6, 23)

If you have wondered about topical creams, lotions, and other cosmetic items, you must know now that gluten must be ingested to affect you. Applying an item to your skin, face, hair, or scalp does not put you at risk for intestinal destruction.

Some celiacs are more sensitive to airborne gluten than others. Because wheat flour does float in the air, a celiac baker will probably have to find another occupation.

Communion wafers are not gluten free. There are some commercially made, but their availability varies by religious denomination. Discuss using a substitute wafer with your minister or priest, or provide your own gluten-free wafer.

Lipstick is considered a gluten culprit at times. One article I read indicated that you would have to eat a carload of it to get enough gluten to bother you. However, some lipsticks do have gluten, and if you reapply your lipstick many times a day because you have been licking your lips, it may be a problem. If you suspect that you are getting gluten from an unknown source, the only way to know for sure if the lipstick that you use has gluten in it is to call the manufacturer. (The ingredients on the label are too small to read.)

Many play dough products are made with wheat flour. There are substitutes that can be used, but young celiac children should avoid this without parental supervision, because they will inevitably put it into their mouths.

Some of the pitfalls people with CD encounter comprise problems with cross-contamination. This was discussed Chapter 8 in relation to the kitchen area and in this chapter in regard to medications, but there are other things to consider. Most grocery stores have areas of bulk foods now. Because you do not know whether the scoop in the candy bin has also been used in the flour bin, or whether the bins have cleaned out between uses, it is best not to utilize the bulk food department. If a store offers pre-packaged bulk foods, you must consider the possibility of cross-contamination. My husband tried to find some chocolate-covered cherries for me as a gift last year. Every candy shop where he inquired stated that they used wheat flour on the work surface to keep the chocolate from sticking.

Some people have concern regarding licking stamps and envelopes. Most dietitians will tell you that you would have to lick many, many stamps or envelopes to get enough gluten to digest it. If you are in doubt, get the self-stick stamps.

Everyone should keep in mind supplies to have on hand in the event of an emergency (tornado, hurricane, or other national disaster). Because gluten-free food is more difficult to obtain, you should plan on having some of the following items available:

Beverages (coffee, tea, powdered milk)
Canned gluten-free foods (including soups and meats, e.g., sardines, tuna, salmon, chicken, etc.)
Dried fruits and nuts
Gluten-free crackers
Protein bars

Some of these (but not canned items) could be safely stored in your freezer and then removed when you need them. That way you will always have the items that you need, fresh. Use up the items on the list so that none become outdated, and replace them regularly. Be sure to keep the items dated and rotate them to ensure freshness.

Some of the other pitfalls that need to be discussed are the fact that it is possible to be obese and have CD. Whether this is because the individual did absorb more calories, or because that individual ate to overcome the symptoms, we do not know. My father weighed two hundred thirty-five pounds when he became ill and died. I believe he had CD. It is even more possible to be overweight after diagnosis. Feeling sick for a long time and then, when the gut starts to heal, feeling so much better, it seems that everything tastes so good, and the newly found gluten-free food is very high in carbohydrates, so one's weight can increase very easily.

Another pitfall in which there is a difference of opinion is that after you eat gluten you will become immediately ill. This is really not always true. Some celiacs do become ill and spend a few or several days getting over the ingestion of gluten. Others are not aware of it and do not realize when gluten is ingested. That is why there are so many "silent celiacs," who may have symptoms of various complaints but no gastrointestinal symptoms. The only way to verify that these folks are gluten intolerant is to check their antibodies on a regular basis. The damage still occurs in the small intestine, even though there are no symptoms.

Silent CD is a real dilemma, because you can have the many conditions that occur because of the damage to your small intestine. These might include, as previously mentioned, osteoporosis, osteopenia, anemia, fibromyalgia, infertility, continuous diarrhea, constipation, bone pain, and other anomalies. The physician might wonder if you have hypochondria because of the myriad complaints that do not fit any particular disease or condition and because you have a high level of anxiety about the illness is indeed a real illness, but because of the presenting symptoms it is difficult to diagnose. Some individuals have severe diarrhea, some have constipation, some are anemic, some have abdominal pain, and others have no symptoms but are screened because a relative has CD, and thus they are diagnosed. These discrepancies make it very difficult if the physician has not read the medical literature and thus is unaware of the symptoms and prevalence of CD.

Some people will say they have "borderline" CD or have a "light case" of it or that they will "outgrow it." According to all of the legitimate literature and research, there is no such thing as any of the above. It would be just like being "a little pregnant." You either have CD or you do not. At this time, the only treatment is a gluten-free diet for life. The only way that gluten induces CD is by ingestion of products containing wheat, barley, or rye. The protein in these grains go through the "gates" in the small intestine, hence the name "leaky gut." The absorption of these proteins throughout the body is the cause of the myriad systemic symptoms.

As mentioned earlier, many times a physician is not aware of the prevalence of CD and therefore does not recognize the symptoms and does not order the appropriate tests. Until just a few years ago, CD was considered a very rare condition. Now that studies have proven that at least one out of every one hundred thirty-three individuals in the United States has the disease, physicians are starting to recognize it as a viable diagnosis. It is up to the celiac community to educate our physicians and communities regarding the symptoms, prevalence, diagnosis, and treatment. CD is not rare and is even more prevalent than HIV.

One of the difficulties with CD is the fact that there are over three hundred different symptoms related to the disease. The following are just a few:

Bloating
Canker sores
Constipation
Delayed growth

Depression
Diarrhea
Discolored teeth
Fatigue
Gas
Headache
Infertility
Itchy rash
Joint pain
Low weight
Numbness
Osteoporosis
Tingling

The wide variety of symptoms explains some of the reasons that CD was so difficult to diagnose prior to the prevalence studies. The prevalence studies that show that only five percent of individuals with CD have been diagnosed bring the diagnosis issue to the forefront and make the health care community more aware of its presence. Because CD is found in ten percent of first-degree relatives (parents, siblings, and children) of individuals with CD, those individuals should be tested for the disease.

The research indicates that about twenty percent of those with Down syndrome have CD, and about twenty percent of individuals with Type 1 diabetes also have it. There are a few other autoimmune conditions that show some prevalence with CD, such as Turner syndrome and Williams syndrome.

Catassi and Fasano from the University of Maryland wrote the following:

Celiac disease (CD) is an autoimmune enteropathy triggered in susceptible individuals by ingestion of gliadin-containing grains. Although the autoimmune process targets mainly the intestinal mucosa, CD can manifest itself with a variety signs and symptoms affecting any organ or tissue. For many years, CD has been underdiagnosed because of poor awareness. However, studies showing a high prevalence of CD in North America, followed by a consensus conference on CD organized by the National Institutes of Health, have fueled a campaign to raise awareness among subspecialists and primary physicians. Nevertheless, guidelines for the diagnosis of CD remain poorly appreciated and many health care professionals remain confused about its proper management. This review is intended to clarify "facts and fantasies" about CD diagnosis. (pp. 466-472)

There are many tests available to be utilized at home for celiac testing. The Celiac Disease Center at Columbia University in New York City has made the following recommendations regarding testing for CD: Of the commercially available serologic tests that aid in the diagnosis of CD, no one test is ideal. Using multiple serologies increases the diagnostic yield. Therefore, in the United States, screening patients in the hospital with possible CD should consist of a panel of the following four serologic tests:

1. Antigliadin antibodies, both immunoglobin A (IgA) and immunoglobin G (IgG)
2. Anti-endomysial antibodies (EMA)-IgA
3. Anti-tissue transglutaminase antibodies (tTG)-IgA
4. Total IgA level

The reasons for the use of the panel of these four tests to detect CD are several. They include selective IgA deficiency, lack of concordance of endomysial antibody and tTG, and the occurrence of seronegative (undetected) CD.

It is still recommended at this time to that one see a physician for a definitive test to determine whether CD is present prior to going on a gluten-free diet.

Some physicians in Argentina have conducted research on testing for CD. They used the deaminated gliadin peptide (DGP) and the tTG test and came to the following conclusion:

> *The DGP/tTG Screen assay could be considered as the best initial test for CD. Combinations of two tests, including a DGP/tTG Screen, might be able to diagnose CD accurately in different clinical scenarios making biopsy avoidable in a high proportion of subjects. (Sugai et al., 2010, pp. 3144-3152)*

It would be wonderful if we could exclude the endoscopy from the initial diagnostic procedure, but at this time that is not an option.

Some radiologists in Italy conducted a study to determine whether there were recognizable changes in a contrast magnetic resonance imaging scan among celiacs on a gluten-free diet, nonceliacs, and untreated celiacs. The results suggested that dynamic evaluation of the bowel wall using contrast-enhanced magnetic resonance imaging can be an effective and reproducible way to show the inflammatory state in CD.

China, India, and Iran are all countries where research is being done on the prevalence, treatment, and screening of CD. This is a good example of the worldwide interest in this disease

A prevalence study conducted in Mexico that showed that one in forty men and one in thirty-five women showed the antibodies for CD. Those are unusually high prevalence rates, and so it will be interesting to follow up on this research.

An article in the *Annual Saudi Medical Journal* stated that restless legs syndrome is a common feature in adult CD.

Each person with CD has a different story to tell:

> *One might have celiac disease (CD) and still be gluten tolerant. I never had the symptoms associated with CD. I did have GERD (gastroesphogeal reflux disease) for many years—due to, according to my [gastroenterologist], a small, sliding hiatal hernia. The GERD symptoms were well controlled with the proton pump*

inhibitor Protonix. After a few years on Protonix, my insurance company wanted tests run to be certain that I didn't have esophageal cancer, as the proton pump inhibitors can mask those symptoms. So, I had an endoscopy. During this procedure, my doctor found and biopsied "dead" villi in my intestine. It was determined that I did, indeed, have CD. Since going on the recommended gluten-free diet—because, it isn't enough just to tolerate gluten—over the years, I have become more sensitive if I happen to stray, either knowingly or by mistake. I am, however, oat tolerant, and the new thinking seems to be that minimally processed oat products may be all right for people who tolerate it. I have also noticed that I am more tolerant of gluten-containing foods if the wheat in question is a "soft" wheat. Wheat varies. Things like cake and delicate pastries are often made with a "softer" wheat than things like bread or pasta. My mother died at age 68 of adenocarcinoma of the lungs after treatment for colorectal cancer. As I think back, I suspect my mother had CD as well. She often had the kinds of symptoms associated with it. My niece and great-niece (a mother and daughter) both have CD. I am a 56-year-old female and was diagnosed in 2002.   BEVERLEY*

The only thing that is of concern regarding this story is that Beverley said that she "has no symptoms if she eats just a small amount of wheat." All of the literature states that any amount can cause an inflammation, which is why all gastroenterologists state that celiacs must be on a gluten-free diet for life.

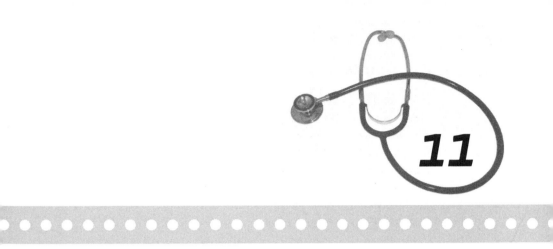

Raising a Gluten-Free Child: Stories From Parents Who Have Been There

We were blessed with a three-week-old [adopted] baby girl who was the most beautiful baby in the world. We named her Lutricia.

She was happy and healthy until about six months old. She would cry often after eating and by the time she was nine months she had diarrhea most of the time. The pediatrician thought she might be lactose intolerant. We took her off milk, but she continued with the diarrhea. After several months of this, we were referred to a gastroenterologist. She did a thorough history and did some lab tests, but she said that she wanted to do an endoscopy.

The follow-up visit was planned for two weeks, but the office called and said "We know you are coming in two weeks, but the labwork has come back and Lutricia has celiac disease (CD). Take her off of bread and wheat products until you come for the next appointment." When I asked about what CD is they assured me that she would be fine and there was nothing to worry about. We did as they asked and found it rather difficult to restrict a sixteen-month-old from eating certain foods. We did notice that her stools were less frequent and she seemed happier within a few days. The doctor had a dietitian on her staff that took about an hour to explain what CD is, what resources are available for gluten-free foods, about a support group that we could attend, the fact that there are genes that must be present to get it, and what kind of research is being done to treat the disease. The alarming thing that we realized is that there is NO treatment but a gluten-free diet. I can write this now because Lutricia is now five years old. She is healthy, happy, and has full knowledge of what she is allowed to eat and what has gluten in it. The interesting thing is, she is adopted. I started having some gastrointestinal symptoms and I was diagnosed with CD. That was the reason that we were unable to conceive. We are all eating gluten free and now I am pregnant with our second child. MARIBETH

After attending a gluten-free support group for several months, I became aware of various parents' attitudes regarding their children with celiac disease (CD). They appeared to be intensively absorbed in, and even defensive at times about, food for their children.

After giving this considerable thought, I concluded that the only way to understand the problems parents face was to discuss it with them. Their answers were unanimous. All parents felt extremely responsible for protecting their children from anything that will make them ill. When a child cannot talk for herself, it is the parent's obvious responsibility to do it for her. The parents I spoke with agreed on the importance of teaching their children, according to the children's age, to make their own decisions.

"I feel like I cannot make any mistakes when feeding or teaching my child, because his life depends on it," said a mother of a six-year-old boy diagnosed with CD.

"I feel the burden of my child's life is on my shoulders," one parent said. "My child's health depends on what they learn from me and their ability to make the right choices for the remainder of their lives."

"Adults with CD can make their own choices, but a child cannot," said a parent of a one-year-old.

"There are so many social, educational, and cultural activities to consider, and my child is almost out of elementary school and does not want me protecting her all the time," a frustrated parent said. "I know I have to let go, but it is so hard. It has become a way of life for me."

Some research indicates that there is a correlation on how long a baby is breastfed and the age of onset of CD. The discussion includes whether an infant should be given solid (complementary) foods before age six months or should at least be started on solid foods by six months of age. Research has indicated that this could possibly give some immunity to, or better tolerance of, gluten.

After my own diagnosis, my grandchildren wanted to make cookies that I could eat. We made chocolate chip cookies according to a traditional non–gluten-free recipe but with gluten-free flour. The first batch covered the entire cookie sheet. The dough had all run together and fell into crumbs when we tried to remove them from the pan. After we got tired of eating crumbs we threw the rest away. We all had a good laugh on that one. From then on, I relied on tried-and-true gluten-free recipes from a gluten-free cookbook. We still make cookies and especially enjoy eating them. All of our cookies have turned out better than our first batch.

Teenagers have their own set of challenges because they are living at a time when they want to exercise their own independence and will question many things that their parents or other in authority say and do. Some teens may feel peer pressure to the extent that they will have a pizza just to prove they can, or because they want to rebel. If they begin to show gastrointestinal symptoms, they will probably realize on their own that they need to stay gluten free. If they are taught, prior to their teenage years, that they need to be responsible for their diet, they will, it is hoped, be compliant.

You should not punish children when they eat something they know they should not eat and, if they are old enough to understand, explain to them the importance of being educated about CD. As a parent you should include your teenager in shopping and cooking and in researching the availability of gluten-free food and supportive peer groups.

Many children are diagnosed before they are two years old. As most parents know, those formative years are so important, and to have a small baby or toddler to protect is different than helping a teenager. But the bottom line is that knowledge of CD and a gluten-free lifestyle as a way of life must be imparted so the child does not feel different or stand out from other children.

Toddlers under age three years can learn that bread, crackers, or cookies that are not gluten free will make them sick. Continuously reaffirm that fruits and vegetables are a good choice. Each time they ask for a fruit or vegetable for a snack, tell them "That is a good choice." The parent who shared this tip said "This puts me in a position to always have celery and carrot sticks soaking in cold water in the refrigerator, as well as sectioned oranges and tangerines. For a special treat I freeze bananas to make smoothies, and I dip bananas in chocolate for a special treat."

Children under age three spend most of their time at home with their caregiver or a babysitter, or at a day care center. Of course, it is going to take a lot of instructions for the day care providers to be continuously alert to the special needs of the child. For instance, play dough and similar items usually contain wheat. It is normal for small children to put things into their mouths, so caregivers need to be especially aware.

Theresa shared some of her experiences with her daughter, Amina. Amina was diagnosed at age three years and is the only celiac in the family. She is now ten but has been taught from age three what she should have and why. She has mistakenly eaten gluten two or three times and became very ill from it. Theresa said that each time Amina knew right away what had happened, and that has made her very careful to follow the diet. Theresa said that she was very determined not to allow Amina's CD to define who she is. Theresa has taught Amina to work with a gluten-free lifestyle so that she can make decisions on her own. Theresa is active in the Gluten-Free Gang, a support group, and participates in all of the activities that will make her daughter feel good about herself and obtain the knowledge she needs to live with the disease.

Theresa said that they prepare all of their meals at home and take them wherever Amina goes. It is important to make sure your child eats only what you prepare. This may be more time consuming than the parent realizes, but the results will be a happier, healthier baby.

Educating all adults with whom the child interacts is absolutely mandatory. Taking the time to educate others is essential to a child's health. Whether attending day care or preschool, going to a friend or relative's home, or attending a birthday party, your child will be constantly at risk of being exposed to gluten. If a child is not being supervised by a parent, anyone who is responsible in the parent's absence needs to be educated as to the importance of the child eating gluten free.

Shawn, whose son Collin is now in college, graciously shared with me their family story, which is a rather typical kind of CD experience.

Collin was diagnosed when he was nine years old. Shawn told me that he is now 19 and is six feet, six inches tall. When asked about his history, she said that as a baby, she breastfed him for about six months.

When Collin was put on formula he was not able to tolerate it, so he was changed to soy formula. At approximately three years of age he had frequent diarrhea and was found to be lactose intolerant. He still continued to have abdominal pain on occasion and in the middle of a meal he would put his fork down and stop eating.

At nine years of age Collin had "stomach flu" followed by severe heartburn. The doctor asked on the next visit how he was feeling, and he answered "I am OK, except for my regular pain." He described it as the pain that he gets when he gets full. The doctor was alarmed at that and referred him to a gastroenterologist. Collin was diagnosed with CD.

Collin did not have growth problems. He was tall for his age and always thin. His food choices included avoiding buns, sandwiches, or cookies while growing up (this was by choice) prior to being gluten free. The most difficult time was during his preteen and teenage years. He did not like to feel different. His mother prepared his lunch every day until he went to high school. They talked to the cafeteria staff so that he could make choices. He apparently cheated on his diet in high school because he did not want to be "different." He said that he knew that he would pay for cheating, and he usually did get sick. His antibody tests are now negative every year, which indicates he is making very good choices by following a gluten-free diet.

Collin's parents are both gluten intolerant but have never been tested for CD. The entire family eats gluten free. Collin is now fully responsible for his food choices, although he has not learned to cook as of yet. His mother told me she had a totally different perspective of CD than Collin. She wanted to protect him in every situation, and he just wanted not to be different.

Elementary school years will be a challenge, because these younger children must eat in a cafeteria and attend parties, Boy or Girl Scouts, children's religious groups, and other activities that take them away from home. Occasionally a relative will say "Oh, just a little bit will not hurt you." If you have read this book, thus far, you realize that a gluten-free diet is for life. *Any* amount of gluten can cause damage and make the child ill. Even if the child has no symptoms, he or she must be taught what foods are allowed on a gluten-free diet. Children also must be taught what is not allowed and why they cannot eat certain foods.

If a child is gluten intolerant and someone insists that he take a food item with gluten, he should simply say "No thank you; I am gluten intolerant." If the person continues to insist, that person probably does not understand. The child should reply "I am very allergic to it, and it will make me sick." Adults' comprehension must be considered as well as children's.

The following story was told to me by the mother of four-year-old Fay.

When Fay was born, we were living in a Florida backwater which had no nearby specialists. We have close friends in the medical field, and one is an excellent pediatrician. I breastfed Fay for fourteen months and we didn't introduce her to solid food until she was almost six months old.

Almost immediately, she had problems. She was already on the slim side, but we paid this no heed because this is a family trait on her father's side. We contended with horrible periodic rashes. Soon after, with our pediatrician's blessing, we toyed with her diet, and after about six months, and a lot of research, it became apparent the problems were related to milk and wheat/gluten.

Milk gave her diarrhea. Wheat/gluten, however, gave her an acidic diarrhea that smelled terrible and literally burned her skin raw (like acid). After so much research, we felt the problem was obvious, and we were not willing to make her suffer through allergy tests and/or the endoscopy necessary to confirm her diagnosis. The fact of the coinciding lactose intolerance led me to conclude

What Nurses Know . . .

Do not punish your child for going off the diet; instead, offer some positive feedback and realize that accidents happen.

she had CD. This has been confirmed by the fact that, after two years on a gluten-free diet, she can now tolerate most dairy products. I would presume her intestine has healed to the extent that she can probably digest it.

Now [that] we're in the New York [City] metro area, we intend to undergo genetic testing as soon as we can afford it. Until then, we know she's thriving on a gluten-free diet and see no reason to question what has been obvious in our case.

How do we deal with it on a daily basis? Despite both of us working full time, we cook everything from scratch. We read every label, and we follow the blogs. We've developed our own rice-flour-based recipes for some of her favorite items, like pancakes and waffles. I could kiss someone at General Mills for their affordable cake and cookie mixes, as well as Chex cereal being gluten free. Her nursery school has a big list of things she can and cannot eat, and she is monitored closely during snack time. We bring our own snacks virtually everywhere and have, thus far, avoided "class parties," which usually revolve around cake and pizza. In the future, I intend to have her bring her own so she can enjoy with everyone—this is what we do for family events as well.

Other than my mom, my family was not very supportive—one of the reasons we moved back to New Jersey from Florida. My brother's wife thought nothing of giving Fay whatever she felt like. (I'll never understand why someone would give a malted candy ball to a sixteen-month-old in any event, as a choking hazard alone.) She once accused me of "making up" CD.

On the other hand, my husband's family is very supportive and makes the effort to avoid gluten-containing foods (my mom-in-law says she's never read so many labels in her life) and, when they can't be avoided, everyone's careful to keep unsafe things out of reach. We all stock up on safe foods she really enjoys: fruits, vegetables, nuts, popcorn. We've only had to make slight adjustments. We have pasta infrequently now, and when we do, she gets her own gluten-free pasta. She's never known anything else, so, fortunately, none of this has been a major transition for her. As *for us, it's balancing her needs with our budget (which is why we don't all eat the special gluten-free foods).*

I have to say that, if my sixteen-year-old daughter had this problem, I would have been lost. Even sixteen years ago, there were so few products available, and what was available was extremely expensive (my friend has a fourteen-year-old who has CD and she lived a nightmare until they figured it out). We were very lucky for this to happen just at a time when celiac awareness was beginning to emerge. I make a point to buy products from companies that make it easy for me by labeling their products "gluten free." Thankfully, the information was out there for us to find and educate ourselves and our doctor, to be frank, who didn't know much about it until he diagnosed Fay. LINDA

Thankfully, Fay found relief; however, according to the specialists who usually prescribe gluten-free diets, testing should always be done before a baby, child, or adult starts adhering to a gluten-free diet.

I was recently in a health food store and noticed a woman with a little girl, about six years old, going through the gluten-free foods. Her name was Kelly, and I asked if she had CD. She said "No; I am wheat and gluten intolerant."

When I inquired if she had been tested, Kelly's mother said that she had not, but had been gluten free for the last two years. "Since Kelly's health had improved, over the last two years, I thought enough time had elapsed to prove she is wheat and gluten intolerant" she said.

I asked if anyone in her family had been tested for CD, and she replied "No." She said a friend had shown her a magazine article and because something seemed to be wrong with Kelly's digestion, she decided to try putting her on a gluten-free diet. Many people today are on a gluten-free diet because of an article they read, a television show they saw, their own volition, or because a friend or relative suggested that a gluten-free diet might help.

What Nurses Know...

Do not start a gluten-free lifestyle without knowing why you are doing it:

CD

Gluten intolerance

Gluten allergy

Medical professionals, including specialists such as internists, gastroenterologists, pediatricians, and allergists, who are most likely to diagnose gluten allergies, gluten intolerance, or CD, all recommend not going on a gluten-free diet without first undergoing medical testing to verify the diagnosis. If a person with CD is off gluten and decides to be tested, the antibodies will not show up. If one starts eating gluten again, the symptoms will return. Gluten-free diets should always be part of your medical records, regardless of the doctor you are currently seeing.

The National Foundation for Celiac Awareness has a wonderful road map that delineates a 504 Plan as part of the Rehabilitation Act of 1973. This plan can be completed by the parents for their child's school. It has all of the necessary information regarding the child, a description of CD, the treatment, an overview of the child's condition, and the goals of the plan. A copy of this plan can be found in the back of this book. If you make a copy of this plan and fill it out, and you can be assured that your child will have a good experience in school. Also available is a document called *Part F Food Allergy Education, Awareness & Reaction Prevention.* It educates the teachers about classroom management and contains information for the school nurse and food services staff as well as guidelines for field trips and any area where food is involved. Teachers have so many responsibilities in order to meet the needs of each child, and these documents help them, not only with your child but also with others.

School lunches are always a concern for every parent. The school lunches are prepared to serve the "average" student. A specific gluten-free diet would probably stretch the school's imagination. The school years are the ideal time to introduce the things that you want your child to have. If schools would serve a basic, gluten-free lunch that included meat, vegetables, brown rice, and fruit it would put to rest the anxiety of the parents and child.

Choose gluten-free foods that are easy to handle, such as finger foods; small meatballs; rice pasta, which now comes in animal shapes; and mini cakes prepared in muffin tins and topped with the child's favorite cheese. Gluten-free wraps, filled with roasted chicken, cheese, and veggies, are one of my family's favorite foods to take on a picnic. Surprise your child with a hot food container in his lunch box, with leftovers from one of his favorite meals. Just picture his eyes when he opens the container. Always try to include at least one fresh fruit and one crunchy vegetable. You can also make (or buy) bean dip to be used with a variety of crackers, vegetables, or a crisp corn tortilla.

If you live in an area that does not have a store with a line of gluten-free products, see the Resources section at the back of this book and go online, where you can find many items to fit any family's needs. Ordering in larger amounts may be optimal because of the shipping costs.

Have fun! Planning to do fun things is almost as much fun as actually doing them. Everyone loves a party, and there is no reason why parents and their child diagnosed with CD should not enjoy a party. There are many ways to have more fun than one can imagine. How about going to camp; attending a gluten-free conference; finding a Web site just for young people with CD; communicating with others your own age via e-mail; going to a support group with kids (and if there is not one close to you, organize one), making delicious, yummy treats to put in the freezer; and even have a surprise with rice bars or fruit roll ups.. Everything does not have to include food, but let's be realistic: Most parties have food.

Chelsea Clinton, the daughter of former President Bill Clinton, apparently is sensitive to gluten and served a gluten-free cake at her wedding. My daughter-in-law also served a gluten-free cake at her wedding that was made from pistachio flour. She does not have CD but assured me that the cake and most of the meal were gluten free. Needless to say, it was very elegant.

Information on camps is available through the Gluten Intolerance Group (http://www.gluten.net) and perhaps other large organizations. These camps provide education for children with CD and allow them to know that there are many other children like themselves. According to an article in the *Journal of Pediatrics*, children who went to a gluten-free camp had an improved state of well-being compared with children who did not go to camp and had been gluten free less than four years. The article indicated that by the end of the study the children who had attended camp reported that they did not now feel different from other kids, and their level of frustration was decreased. Self-esteem is one of the most precious gifts a child could receive. Start now to find out where the closest camp can be found and, if money is an issue, inquire about scholarships. A gluten-free camp would be a great morale booster for any child.

The national celiac meetings usually have separate sessions for different age groups. They are all very informative and offer new and varied ideas for helping children make good choices. The instructors use unusual fun techniques for reading labels, choosing foods, and educating others. These meetings are well worth attending and always offer up-to-date information and the latest ongoing research.

Some children will ask if they can chew gum. Amy Ratner wrote a detailed article for *Gluten-Free Living* about how she had investigated the makers of chewing gum. Her conclusion was that worrying about gluten in gum seems needless.

There are many wonderful cookbooks and storybooks for children with CD, gluten intolerance, or gluten allergies (see the Resources section at the back of this book). Children who get involved in recipes and stories at an early age will be much more accepting of their restricted diet. It will become their second nature. There are many items that are made gluten free and marketed just for children, including snack bars, cereals, frozen entrees (e.g., pizza, chicken nuggets, breakfast items), fruit bars, cookies, and many more. These items may be more expensive, but they will give you options and provide ideas regarding what is available and things you can make at home.

There are several groups that are targeted specifically toward children with CD. One is Raising Our Celiac Kids (ROCK), a support group for children founded by Danna Korn (see http://www.celiac.com/articles/563/1/ROCK-Raising-Our-Celiac-Kids--National-Celiac-Disease-Support-Group/Page1.html). There are currently about sixty-five ROCK chapters in the United States. Korn presents a positive approach to youth as well as to adults. The following are some of the ideas she elaborates on at the URL just provided:

- Finding fun gluten-free treats for kids
- Menu ideas for school lunches, quick dinners, and sports snacks
- Helping kids take responsibility for reading labels, cooking, and planning/preparing food
- How to prepare for unexpected birthday parties and food-oriented activities at school, church, and elsewhere
- How to safely include kids on Halloween, Easter, and other special days
- Educating day care providers and teachers without burdening them
- Dealing with grandparents, babysitters, and "helpful" friends who offer gluten-containing foods to kids
- Ensuring that your children won't cheat on the gluten-free diet, and what to do when they do
- Sending kids away to camp, friends' houses, and other times when the parents are not around to help
- The psychological impact of growing up with CD (peer pressure, teenage years, and more)
- Safe and forbidden ingredients and additives

Korn has written many books and articles specifically dealing with children and CD. She is also a national speaker regarding gluten intolerance and remains active in the ROCK support groups. Her stories are delightful, and parents will probably identify with at least one concept in each of her stories or articles.

It is only normal for parents to want to protect their children; however, if children are overprotected it is difficult for them to accept responsibility, because everything is being done for them. Encouragement and faith will help a child make the right decisions and will go much further than criticism. If a child makes the wrong decision, parents, instead of reacting out of anger or disgust, should ask "Why did you make that decision?" This opens the door for dialogue. When dealing with something as crucial as a child's self-esteem and children's ability to make the right decisions regarding their health for the rest of their lives, we must gently massage the ground around them and not use a bulldozer. Always remember to encourage individual responsibility. Always ask your child "What is the right choice?" so when she is old enough to go places on her own she will automatically ask herself this question. Life is not just a list of rules about what to eat and what not to eat. Use positive affirmations, and try not to criticize. If we expect children to make the right decisions, they will try to live up to our expectations. Every child wants acceptance from a parent; it doesn't matter how old or young the child is. Parents' attitudes have a direct effect on their children. The parent must decide to be the adult. Always make the decision to act with intelligence, and never react with emotion. Children learn how to act, react, and make the right decisions from the teaching of concerned parents. Remember, just do your best and don't take life too seriously. Take time to have fun, be happy, and laugh.

Dining Out: Safely and Enjoyably

Dining out was a traumatic experience after being diagnosed with celiac disease (CD). I recall going to a restaurant about thirteen years ago, reading the menu, and then, with tears rolling down my cheeks, not knowing where to start. Eating gluten free was rare at that time and very few people had heard of it. Fortunately, most culinary arts schools now teach the gluten-free diet as part of the curriculum. After that first try, I decided that CD was not going to limit me from doing anything that I wanted to do. I knew that I had to change my attitude. I was determined to learn how to express myself so I could get what I wanted and needed. My husband and I are both retired and enjoy traveling. Consequently, it is imperative that I am able to eat anywhere. I can honestly say that this has worked. There are very few restaurants where I will not at least try to find something that is gluten free. GLADYS

Everyone differs as to how they approach a dining experience. If you are going to an elegant restaurant, then you can be sure that the chef will be very accommodating. In fact, there is a lovely Italian restaurant in our area that has a Sunday buffet. Our family went there after church. The waitress checked as to whether the glaze on the petite filets was gluten free. She proceeded to bring me two filets without any glaze. There was plenty of fresh fruit, salads, and other acceptable dishes, which made a wonderful meal. Of course, dessert and pasta are out, but that is not so bad when everything else is gluten free and so good. This sort of experience is not uncommon in more expensive restaurants.

Family-style restaurants usually fry all their foods in the same oil as their breaded items, so be sure to check about french fries, or just skip the fries. The grill will not be gluten free if the kitchen staff cook pancakes or sandwiches on the same grill as the other foods. Sometimes it is better just to order a salad or breakfast food because you can order eggs and bacon and omit the toast. The other option, to prevent contamination, is to ask that meat be prepared on a piece of foil on the grill. Throughout this book I have stressed the importance of a good attitude in approaching a gluten-free lifestyle. This is one of those times. Never let the place or experience keep you from eating out. You will most likely be able to find something on the menu that will be safe. Check ahead of time, and if there really is nothing you can eat at a particular restaurant, go ahead and meet your friends there and, if the local or state food codes do not prohibit this, take your own food, otherwise just order and beverage and a salad.

Read the menu carefully. Does a soup look safe? How about lentil, bean, or vegetable soup? Pick out three items that sound good and ask the server to check whether they are gluten free. They can do that and let you know what is available. Just make sure they know this includes wheat, barley, and rye. I have never had one server refuse to check for me. Sometimes they must consult the manager, but that is fine. The manager wants customers to return; consequently, they will usually go beyond the call of duty to honor patron requests.

What Nurses Know...

Check the Web sites of restaurants for a gluten-free menu. You might be surprised to learn how many have them available now.

Many restaurants have gluten-free menus and/or list the gluten-free items on their Web sites. Fast food places were the first to offer a gluten-free list on their Web sites. It is extremely important to check before ordering french fries. If the coated chicken nuggets are cooked in the same oil as the fries, then the oil is contaminated with gluten. Some Wendy's and McDonald's do not use the same oil, but every restaurant is different. As a result, it is mandatory to always ask. Wendy's baked potato, Frosty, salad, or a burger without the bun is always a quick meal. Again, you can always check the Web site before going to be sure. Even Subway will now prepare a breakfast sandwich wrapped in an egg, or a regular sandwich can be wrapped in a large piece of lettuce.

Patty was willing to share her experiences with her son and husband, who eat gluten free, and another son who has eosinophilic esophagitis and for many years had a feeding tube for nourishment.

Patty said that she and her family have traveled worldwide and they are most comfortable going back to restaurants where they have been treated best. If a chef in a hotel was able to meet their needs, they plan on going back to that hotel. She stated that they never eat in fast food restaurants but will always go back to a restaurant that they know and one that knows them. She said when she sent her sons to preschool, kindergarten, and first grade, she was a volunteer and was always there on the first day with a signed letter in hand detailing what the school needed to know. She would role play with her sons using medical terms, foods they were allowed to have, and what they needed to know

What Nurses Know...

Eosinophilic esophagitis is an inflammatory condition in which the wall of the esophagus becomes filled with large numbers of eosinophils, a type of white blood cell.

about their conditions so they could talk to an adult with knowledge and poise.

When one of her sons went to band camp, Patty said she did not say "He needs this kind of diet." She got a hotel room, where she took boxes and coolers full of food, and she took her son back to the hotel to do the tube feedings. He did not miss any practice and was able to participate in band camp. She said if the camp leaders had been approached with her son's needs they would have been overwhelmed and likely would not have wanted to assume the responsibility. Prearranging for those needs allowed her son to participate and not feel isolated or different.

Patty recommends planning six months ahead when traveling. Plan to pack at least one week worth of dry gluten-free foods, know where the food markets are located, and always ask for a refrigerator in the hotel room.

Preparing for college at Indiana University was a challenge for Patty and her family. They started six months ahead. They went to the school and met with the dining hall managers, chefs, and administrators. She had in writing a list, signed by her son's physician, of all the gluten-free items that her son was allowed to eat. The dining hall staff had a shelf in the kitchen designated with her son's name on it, and they knew exactly what to prepare for him. He had a refrigerator in his dorm room, and Patty brought an eight-week supply of food for him. Patty believes she has empowered her children with knowledge, enabling them to be assertive or receptive in doing whatever is necessary to fulfill their dietary needs.

A restaurant card, which tells the server exactly what you need, is one option when you are dining out. **(These cards are commercially available, although support groups provide them as well.)** The disadvantages of these cards are that they have to be wordy to be effective, and the restaurant may not want the legal responsibility of guaranteeing a gluten-free meal. They do not want you to get sick, and you do not want to get sick. In presenting restaurant cards to busy servers, I found that they did not have the time to read it, and sometimes it caused more problems than results.

A popular TV personality who eats gluten free states that she insists on restaurants preparing her food in separate pans and skillets. Her demands make it a nightmare for the chefs and servers. Yes, we must be extremely careful in our food choices. You would not want to choose something that is obviously full of gluten. You know that you can have a salad with no croutons and that most salad dressings are gluten free. Meat can be ordered broiled or grilled on a piece of aluminum, without sauce. Vegetables can usually be ordered steamed. Baked potatoes are always an option. So you see, by reading the menu carefully, you can order by being specific and get what you need to stay gluten free without making unreasonable demands on the restaurant staff.

It is so important to tell the server immediately that you cannot eat wheat, barley, or rye. Be very specific, and if they make a mistake, it is not your fault. However, if one is not clear about one's needs and the restaurant makes a mistake, it is not the restaurant's fault. When you order a steak or prime rib, be specific

What Nurses Know...

Read menus carefully and choose a few items that sound good to you; then ask the server to determine whether they can be prepared gluten free.

What Nurses Know...

Remember, wheat is used to make au jus, so if you order prime rib tell your server not to include au jus.

and tell them "No bread under the meat." When you order a salad, tell them "No croutons on the salad." We do not want to be argumentative over our food, but it is in fact a medical necessity to be gluten free. That is why it is so important to be very explicit. The more something is said the easier it becomes to say it again, so practice at home and soon the words will roll off your tongue.

When going to a banquet, special invitation dinner, wedding, or some other formal social occasion, it is imperative, when returning the response card, that you write in that it is medically necessary that you eat a gluten-free meal. When you arrive at the event, you do not need to talk with anyone but your server about your meal; just state that you ordered a gluten-free meal and explain where you will be sitting. If the staff state that they were not expecting you, tell them that the gluten-free meal request was on your response card and that it is essential for you to have a gluten-free meal. You will find that they are most always accommodating to meet those needs, but it is helpful if they know it ahead of time.

The Gluten-Free Gang of central Ohio has a web site (http://www.glutenfreegang.org) with a list of all local (and some national) restaurants that have gluten-free menus. It is helpful to just check there if you are in doubt, or you can consult your local CD support group (see the Resources section at the back of this book) or the restaurant's Web site.

What is more satisfying than going to an Outback Steakhouse restaurant, ordering a meal that is gluten free from a real gluten-free menu, and then topping it off with a "Thunder From Down Under?" Wow, that is really heaven.

What Nurses Know...

When going to a reservation-only dining event, make sure at the time you make your reservation that you indicate that you require a gluten-free meal. When you arrive, tell your server that you have ordered a gluten-free meal and indicate where you are sitting.

Teresa is a member of the Gluten-Free Gang but lives in a small town with fewer resources than a large urban area. Her daughter, Alissa, is seventeen years old and was diagnosed with CD about one and a half years ago:

We have struggled with this disease for some time, not knowing what was wrong with her. We went years thinking as parents this was "all in her head," since every doctor had no answers for us. We went from doctor to doctor with diagnoses from "It is in her head" to she "has [attention-deficit/hyperactivity disorder]," and they put her on medicine for it. I, as the parent, said no more on that one. They diagnosed her with anxiety, depression, gastric bowel syndrome. They even went so far as making us do rub-downs on her body to eliminate "all the yuck out of her." Finally, our doctor sent her to the physician assistant. She said, "We are going to run any and all tests so we can figure this out." Well, sure enough, we finally got an answer. The blood test showed it, and the [endoscopy] proved that she had CD. We have been on a really emotional roller coaster with this, and of course now, with challenges of food.

This August we went to Disney World in Florida, and of course we were thinking we were just going to have her eat scrambled eggs, hamburgers with no bun, and salad. Much to our surprise Disney World has a gluten-free menu!

I had e-mailed them before our trip asking if they do and within twenty-four hours I had an e-mail back of every restaurant at Disney that serves gluten-free food and what there is to eat there. They broke it down for us for each place: Magic Kingdom, water parks, Animal Kingdom, Hollywood Studios, EPCOT, and all the resorts that serve food. It was the easiest experience I have dealt with. Every place that we went in we told them we needed a gluten-free menu. A chef would come out and talk to [Alissa] and tell her what she could and could not eat and tell her how he or she cooks the food. At Crystal Palace, a character buffet, the chef came out and brought her gluten-free rolls and butter and then took her to the buffet and pointed out everything that she was allowed to eat. They would go into the kitchen for her and make sure they got her meal ready. I have never been so happy in my life at the "happiest place on earth." It was the first vacation that we have been where we didn't cook the food and Alissa didn't have a stomachache. What a relaxing vacation. And the best part was the chicken fingers were to die for. They tasted like ours. The pizza was awesome. The waffles and pancakes were super. I really can't think of anything she didn't like. The rolls were even good. Well, I do take that back. There was a brownie at one of the restaurants that wasn't very good, but heck, she had so much good food she didn't care so much about the brownie.   TERESA

That was certainly a wonderful vacation that made many good memories. That is what dining out and traveling should be about, making memories.

Potlucks are usually a challenge for anyone eating gluten free. It is a good idea if you take something that you know is gluten free. Explain to whoever is in charge that you cannot take the chance of contamination of foods through utensil transfer and that you request to go to the front of the line. Most people will understand and be willing to accommodate you. You can then have some of what you brought and any plain vegetables, fruits, and salads. You may take your own dessert, or even your own meal, if you are more comfortable. The purpose of most potlucks is for the fellowship and you do not want to miss that.

In the past five years, I have been amazed at how many more restaurants are willing to identify what is gluten free. If you know that you are going to a fast food place, look it up on the Web so you will know which menu items you can have. Many children's groups (e.g., soccer teams) have treats and/or go to places after their team wins. Parents need to be involved with that, so be prepared to tell your child ahead of time what is allowed, or provide a separate snack for the child.

In Chapter 11 I mentioned Danna Korn, founder of the support group Raising Our Celiac Kids and provider of some great youth-oriented resources, including books and the Web site http://www.celiackids.com. The following excerpt is from an article by Korn entitled "Venturing Out of the House: Restaurant Realities":

It's been said that the best offense is a good defense, which probably applies to restaurant excursions as well as it does to the football field. I'm not encouraging you to be offensive; in fact, quite the opposite. It's not, after all, the waiters' or chefs' responsibility to accommodate your diet. If they do, be prepared to leave a big tip, because their job descriptions definitely do not include understanding the intricacies of this diet. Nor should you fill them in on all the minutiae surrounding the diet.

A brief education is all they should need, because you should already have narrowed down the choices on the menu that look as though they might be safe, or at least may be prepared in a way that would make them safe. It's okay to ask that your food be prepared in a special manner— people do that all the time even when they are not on a special diet.

Most important, you need to be aware of specific foods and ingredients to avoid when eating out. Some things are more likely to be okay than others, and you should make it easier on yourself by choosing items that are more likely to be wheat-free/gluten-free.

It is obvious that one of your top priorities should be educating yourself and the community about living a gluten-free lifestyle. Knowledge empowers you to be assertive to get what you need to be healthy.

My mom usually orders for me when we go out to eat because I don't know how to do it. I look at the kids menu and she orders for me. I never deviate from eating gluten free. I don't even if they say it is okay. I eat the same things all the time. Chicken salad, sometimes plain hamburger.

I am continually invited to birthday parties. My good friend's mom gets ice cream for me or cupcakes at Whole Foods. They always offer me fruit or if they don't have gluten-free pizza, just salad, corn, or chicken. My biggest challenge is when people eat food I can't have. I know there is always something they are eating I cannot eat. I don't care that much because I don't want to get sick.

This year in school my teachers said no food is to be brought into class for birthdays because some kids can't participate and it is not fair for them to sit and watch. Kids must bring a small gift like pencils or buy a book for the library. The best thing about being a celiac is that I don't have to do table washing at school because the towel has wheat on it. GRACIE

Well, seven-year-old Gracie does get out of the table washing. She did a good job of making us realize that she does not go off her diet because she does not want to get sick. It is great to hear how such a young child is able to deal with a gluten-free lifestyle.

Attitude is still very important when making a decision to eat out. Yes, the first time may be hard, but after that you should decide to be assertive and in control so that you get what you need. If you need to carry a restaurant card, that is fine. If you need to carry a letter signed by your doctor, that too is acceptable. If you are comfortable discussing your needs with the restaurant manager, that's great. If after asking your server for what you need you get a blank stare, you know that you will have to go a step further and ask for a chef or a manager. Many of the national chain restaurants are sent food preprepared so that the local facility has no say about ingredients. If that is the case, you will know that is not a friendly gluten-free place.

Some families like to go out to eat often; others prefer to dine out only on special occasions. If you are going out for a special occasion, call ahead and make sure that you can talk to someone who can assure you that your meal will be gluten free. Never call or go out to eat during busy mealtimes; that is when mistakes happen, and you will be disappointed. Call in the morning or midafternoon and, if possible, make your reservation for whatever time the staff tell you is the least busy. One of the worst experiences can happen when the kitchen is very busy and the workers are trying to meet everyone's needs at once.

Frederick took his wife, Jasmine, out to a Hilton Hotel restaurant for their anniversary. They went at 5:00 p.m. and were the only ones in the restaurant. The chef came to their table and assured Jasmine that the meal she had ordered could be made gluten free. After dinner the chef returned to see how everything was and even shared with them a risotto recipe that was wonderful. Frederick and Jasmine left the restaurant about 6:30 p.m., and it still was not busy, so they decided they had picked a good time. Sometimes it is better to save money for a special dinner at an upscale restaurant than to go to less expensive place that does not have a clue what you mean by "gluten free."

There are a few other ways to make your dining out more enjoyable. If you go to an Italian restaurant and you know that they serve oil with herbs for dipping, ask for a separate dish and, with management approval, take your own bread so that you can dip also. Yum! Some Italian restaurants now have gluten-free menus.

If you are invited to an event by an acquaintance with whom you are not really familiar, ask what he or she will be serving, and take your own casserole or main dish so that the hostess does not have to go to any trouble. Explain your situation and offer to also take dessert. Another option is to give your friends a list of the things that you are allowed to have. They can then call you if they have a question but it likely will make them feel better to know they can provide a gluten-free meal for you.

We always expect families to accept our problems and learn the details of something like a gluten-free diet. I'm sorry to disappoint you, but there will be family members who do not understand or are not interested in learning about eating gluten free. There is only one other disease that requires a special diet, and that is diabetes mellitus. Individuals with diabetes can quietly accept or reject foods without any issues. Individuals who are gluten intolerant cannot. You must know what is in an item before you will know whether it is safe. It is not worth becoming ill at the expense of a family member who does not understand. We are all aware that if there is a pill to correct it, advertising would flood the TV screens and everyone would know about gluten intolerance. However, there is not; the only lifetime treatment is to eat gluten free.

Georgia and her family were invited to a relative's for Thanksgiving dinner. Georgia explained that she could not eat the turkey if it had regular bread stuffing, so she offered to make the stuffing. When they got to the dinner, the turkey had been stuffed with regular bread. All of the sauces had been thickened with flour, and all of the desserts were made with wheat flour. Georgia was very disappointed and had trouble not showing her emotions because she was not sure what she was going to eat. Georgia was polite and explained to the hostess (her sister-in-law) that, if she wished, Georgia could give her a list of the things that she was allowed for the next get-together. Some of the other family members wanted a list too. Georgia obviously could eat only the stuffing and the cranberry sauce she had brought. The next family event went much better because Georgia had provided each member with her list, and they were much more aware of reading labels and how to prepare gluten-free foods. This is an example of the learning curve for living a gluten-free lifestyle. It has been said before that knowledge is power; that is so true. The more that we educate those around us, the easier it will be for us now and for all the gluten-intolerant individuals coming after us.

One family recounted to me that they had a completely gluten-free meal for Thanksgiving. One daughter brought gluten-free stuffing and cranberry sauce. The turkey was roasted with vegetables inside. The other vegetables were all prepared gluten free. Another daughter brought gluten-free pumpkin and apple pies. A son brought gluten-free oyster stuffing and pecan pie. A daughter-in-law brought a gluten-free cheesecake. There also was a relish plate with fresh vegetables, shrimp cocktail, and remake made with gluten-free soy sauce as appetizers. This family had a feast, and it was all gluten free, so it was enjoyed by all.

The parents of a celiac child perceive dining out quite differently than an adult without CD. The adult learns to pull him- or herself up by the bootstraps and make the best of it. Children taught from the time that they are diagnosed what is acceptable to eat and, if the parents are present, that is not a problem. It is the emotional aspect that overshadows the parent who is trying to protect a child. I am certain that, after protecting the child for several years, it becomes a habit that is difficult to change and allow the child to make his choices. As Gracie described earlier in this chapter, she stays on the diet so that she does not get sick.

The Americans With Disabilities Act of 1990 applies to schools that receive any federal funding. Because a gluten-free diet is the only treatment for CD, federally funded schools must make provisions for gluten-free meals for students. However, school kitchen staff are not professionally trained chefs, and they must be educated and assisted until the parents are comfortable with the situation. Successful implementation of gluten-free food for a student requires involvement by means of volunteering, frequent visits, and lots of cooperation. At least one parent needs to make that commitment, or there is the chance that the child will not get the needed diet.

Jack took his wife out for dinner after a busy day. His wife told the waitress that she had CD, and the waitress smiled and said "OK." The chef came to the table and introduced himself and stated that he also had CD as well as two children who had it. He also had a child that was on a gluten-free and casein-free diet and thus he was very familiar with what she could have. She made a few choices—a Caesar salad, prime rib, and "smashed" potatoes—and he said that he could prepare those items gluten free without any difficulty. Poor Jack was so involved in the conversation that he lost his appetite and ordered a club sandwich. The sad thing about this story is that the restaurant made a corporate decision that they did not want the legal liability of stating that anything is gluten free. Jack's wife promptly wrote them a letter telling them how wonderful her meal was and encouraged the entire corporation to step out and serve the three million gluten-intolerant people who need to eat gluten free. In fact, she told them, they already had an employee on board who could make that happen.

What Nurses Know . . .

We need to be cognizant of the family members and friends who have to sit and listen each and every time we go out to eat. Gluten-free eating can interfere with interpersonal relationships. Tell your friends or family about your eating issues beforehand so they can either help pick a spot that would work for all of you or can be patient while you try to get the right type of food for you.

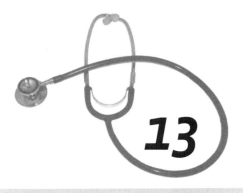

13

Travel Tips

Robin (a local travel agent) thought a cruise would suit my yen to travel and introduced me to Norwegian Cruise Lines. My first trip by myself was to the Caribbean.

Naturally, one of my biggest concerns was "What will I be able to eat?" After making the cruise arrangements, a representative from the food department of the cruise lines called me to discuss my gluten-free diet. Upon my arrival, there was a bowl of fresh fruit waiting for me in my cabin along with instructions regarding my gluten-free meals. As dinner hour approached, I got antsy and reported to the maître d' for my instructions to find he had already received notification of my dietary needs. He assured me that he would have everything under control. Since I was alone, each night the headwaiter found me great dinner companions.

The maître d' certainly did his job. Each night in the main dining room, I would arrive and be greeted with what I could eat on the menu. In many cases, the chef made special gluten-free desserts. Bravo for going above and beyond what I expected.

Shore excursions were somewhat of a challenge. If the group that I was in was having lunch ashore, I contacted the Shore Excursion office to determine if anything was gluten free.

My experience with cruising was flawless; however, I do not have a positive statement to make about my airline travel. Airline food (or lack of it) is the fodder for comedian's monologues. I have traveled on many different airlines. On flights where meals were served, getting a gluten-free meal is a roll of the dice, even when you call ahead. They serve snacks of peanuts, pretzels, or cookies. I have learned to carry gluten-free cookies, rice crackers, and gluten-free pretzels in my carry-on luggage. I found that fruit is not the smartest thing to bring as it ends up in the trash when you go through security.

Another thing to remember when traveling is always watch out for what you drink. I had a reaction to a mai tai in Hawaii. The rum is gluten free, but I failed to ask the bartender what constituted [the rest of the ingredients in] the special drink at the hotel. MARY

Mary is remarkable. She is a very hard worker and active in the Gluten-Free Gang, a support group based in central Ohio. She helps wherever and whenever she is needed. She is also an advocate to educate others and make sure that every one that she meets understands and knows about celiac disease (CD) and the necessity of a gluten-free diet for the gluten intolerant.

Some individuals with gluten intolerance may be reluctant to go on a cruise. If you approach a cruise in the same manner that you approach the rest of dining out opportunities, you will find that preparation helps. First, tell your travel agent you must eat gluten free and offer a physician's statement describing that this is a medical necessity. You will be told when you arrive on board to talk to the maître d'. You can do that at the next meal. When you arrive, there is usually a buffet waiting. This is an opportunity to eat fresh fruits, vegetables, and maybe one of your carry-on snacks. Many of the buffet items will be in a sauce or obviously full of gluten, and you'll know what to avoid. You can try to ask one of the chefs if there is wheat in any particular item, but you may have trouble getting an answer at the buffet because the cruise staff are usually very busy, and some do not speak English.

At dinnertime, ask for the maître d' if you have not talked to him or her previously. The maître d' will either go over the menu with you or assign a headwaiter, who will explain what is gluten free on the menu for that evening and will come to your table on subsequent evenings, and show you the menu for the next day, and tell you what the chef recommends for someone on a gluten-free diet.

As you know, most desserts are not gluten free. On my last cruise, the chef made a wonderful dessert surprise every night that included crème brûlée, tiramisu, and chocolate lava cake. It makes me salivate just writing about the food on that cruise. I was able to pick from the menu, an appetizer, soup, entrée (sometimes two), vegetables, cheese, and bread (if I chose). They did have gluten-free cookies and bread and would make gluten-free pancakes if ordered the day before. The headwaiter talked to the chef who prepared the meal and would reassure me each day that my food was gluten free. I ordered some French toast that was delicious.

Of course, it is impossible to promise that your cruise would be this good, but after going on many cruises and having only one be not so good, I really recommend cruising and believe the cruise lines make an honest effort to accommodate the gluten-free lifestyle. A cruise is a wonderful vacation.

Traveling abroad can be challenging for people on a gluten-free diet, but traveling to a relative's house can be just as much of a challenge.

Traveling to relative's homes has gotten easier the past several years, once everyone was made aware of what CD is and what is a gluten-free diet. Most of my relatives complied. My sister in law in Buffalo [immerses] herself in gluten-free shopping and cooking every time I visit. Even my son-in-law, whom I visited this summer in Italy, had some interesting foods he prepared that were gluten free. Being in Italy with all that pasta was challenging. I was so glad that my grandson could speak fluent Italian. He was able to translate the menu and question the server and chef about my food.

Before I left for Italy, I sent a large box of gluten-free food to my daughter's home in Sicily. It was a good thing that I did. The Navy commissary had very little in the way of gluten-free foods. They carried Rice and Corn Chex, and one brand of crackers that I could have. My box sure came in handy.

Bob and Ruth Levy have a travel group called "Bob and Ruth's Gluten-Free Dining and Travel [Club]." This past winter, I traveled with them to Cancun, Mexico. Bob made sure that our chef, Mauricio, had wonderful desserts and foods that most of us had not tasted in a long time. The food was awesome, and I was impressed with the details that went into our meals. Bob and Ruth had a meeting upon our arrival, and he went around the room questioning us if there was any particular food we were craving. I mentioned onion rings. When the onion rings were brought out on our last night, Mauricio gave me a whole plate full of these delicious and heartburn-producing meal accompaniments. Wow, was I impressed; they were awesome!

I have not found a place yet where I cannot get a steak. This meat is something that I can find at most foreign restaurants. I guess that I am going to have to say "No gluten, no wheat flour" in a few more languages. MARY

The best thing you can do for yourself when traveling is always carry snacks or enough food to last until you reach your destination. Most airlines do not serve meals; unless the flight is a very long one they just provide snacks. Prepare several gluten-free

What Nurses Know...

The following are some suggested snacks to pack while traveling: nuts, dried fruit, gluten-free pretzels, gluten-free crackers with peanut butter, fruit roll-ups. Bring enough so that if the unexpected happens you are prepared.

snack bags for traveling, so that you will always have something that you want.

Patty's husband and son are both gluten intolerant, and she shared with me her family's method of coping with food while traveling. She said that whenever they travel they always take a large suitcase with dry gluten-free food. When they arrive at their destination they find the closest market so they can get perishables and other food items. They always get a hotel room with a refrigerator so they can get milk, fruit, and other things they will need in order to avoid fast food or take a chance on a restaurant they do not know.

I am a choreographer/teacher/adjudicator in the wonderful world of dance. I travel quite a bit and really had to change my travel style after being diagnosed with CD in April of 2009. I am very dedicated to living my life gluten free. The payoff has been tremendous, and I feel better at the age of 41 than I did at age 31!

Las Vegas—I was judging a national dance competition in Las Vegas at the MGM Grand. Happy to report that restaurants Emeril's, Rainforest Cafe, Diego, and Wolfgang Puck at the MGM Grand all had fantastic gluten-free menus!! The general manager at Emeril's follows a gluten-free diet so he really knew what he was talking about! Wolfgang Puck has a chicken marsala with polenta and asparagus to die for! The MGM Grand also placed a mini-refrigerator in my room within twenty minutes after my request. I easily kept fruit, water, and snacks in my room.

New York City—Risotteria is a gluten-free and vegetarian Italian restaurant and bakery. They had wonderful gluten-free risotto, breadsticks, pizza, panini, breads and many other yummy baked goods. At S'MAC I had a skillet full of gluten-free hamburger macaroni and cheese. I had my first gluten-free cheeseburger, outside of my home, at Blooms Deli. It came complete with a gluten-free bun and gluten-free french fries. It was a little bit of heaven! Babycakes Bakery…wow! If I had this bakery near my home, I just might be addicted to their cupcakes! Ruby Foo's had delicious Asian food including gluten-free soy sauce.

Chicago—Weber Grill had a great gluten-free menu and out of this world delicious steaks. I was a professional dancer in Chicago for several years and adore Chicago deep-dish pizza. After some research I found Lou Malnati's had a crustless pizza, so I gave it a try. My friends all had deep-dish pizza from another pizzeria delivered and I had Malnati's delivered. I was so pleasantly surprised as I sunk my teeth into the cheesy pizza that had a crust made of sausage! I know sausage crust sounds crazy, and it is not low calorie, but it was fantastic! I did not feel a bit deprived and the flavors were delicious!

Myrtle Beach—Went with my husband and daughter. Cheeseburger in Paradise, Dairy Queen, River City Cafe, Pier 14 were all great. However, I made a very poor judgment on the last day we were there. My daughter and her friend really wanted to go to [the International House of Pancakes] on the morning we were headed home. So we did. I spoke with the server and the general manager, even showing them my "Triumph Dining Restaurant" gluten-free card. I ordered a veggie omelet and I thought I covered all the bases. I got about a quarter of the way through breakfast and I ran like lightning to the restrooms. I was very sick the rest of the day, and it was our "driving home day." I wish I would have stuck to my power bar and coffee, which is what I usually do if they do not have a gluten-free breakfast menu. TIFFANY

Tiffany would make a good traveling partner because she certainly knows the restaurants in the towns she frequents. She is

What Nurses Know...

Enjoy the journey while traveling. Plan ahead and pack your snacks.

very realistic about the outcomes of taking chances. Once you become more comfortable in making choices when you eat out, you will find there are fewer and fewer times that you become sick.

People who like to camp might find some new and different ideas in the following excerpt from an article entitled "Gluten-Free Camping," by Destiny Stone, which is used by permission of www.celiac.com:

Camping is supposed to be relaxing and fun. Most people camp to escape the monotony of the daily rut, and to get back to the basics. Eating gluten-free while camping is really easy, once you know what to bring and what to avoid.

Camping trips usually consist of the same easy to prepare foods. Chili, pasta, canned soups, hot chocolate, sandwiches, hot cereal, trail mix and s'mores are the high-lights of most camping meals. (Even the graham crackers can be gluten free.) In fact, many gluten-free foods, already produced, can be used for camping trips. Anything canned or boxed that you normally enjoy at home, can typically be converted to camping food.

It is important to eat the perishable foods first. A camping trip lasting for more than one night can render perishable foods inedible. That's why it's important to eat refrigerated food on the first day or two, and save the shelf-stable food for the remainder of the trip. Store perishables in a cooler with plenty of ice and/or cold packs. To grill gluten-free food, avoid gluten contamination by using a grill from home. Using the grill provided at the camping site is possible, but using aluminum foil or a pan as a buffer will keep food away from gluten contamination. There are even special racks with ridges that can be placed on the grill and will keep food from touching the grill.

Some individuals' travel plans include a resort where you stay for a given number of days. April Baxter and her husband went to the Bahamas, and she described her story in the following excerpt (used with the permission of www.celiac.com) from her article "Gluten-Free Travel to Nassau, Bahamas." She was a celiac for ten years prior to this trip:

My husband and I recently returned from a trip to the Sandals Royal Bahamian Resort in Nassau, Bahamas. What a wonderful experience! The resort itself was beautiful but the people working there made the vacation special. Prior to our arrival, I contacted the General Manager, Jeremy Mutton, advising him of my dietary requirements. He promptly responded that I would be taken care of without any problems and had informed the appropriate staff.

Upon our arrival, I was greeted by the Executive Sous Chef, Seanette Brice, and the food/Beverage Manager, Sieon Wintz, who catered to all my dietary needs. I was so impressed by their knowledge of celiac disease and how they took the necessary precautions in having all of my meals prepared. There are 9 or 10 restaurants on the property—most of them we dined at and they all were aware of my gluten free needs—the chefs would actually come out to speak with me prior to each meal—they often made a little something extra for my plate. The Italian Restaurant carried gluten free pasta; the pizzeria on the beach had a special pizza made for me with no cross-contamination; French fries were made in a dedicated fryer; desserts were made especially for me. Fresh fruit was plentiful, as well, every day. All meals/snacks were excellent. Seanette even offered to pack me a lunch the day we went into town to shop!

I highly recommend visiting this resort for a relaxing, gluten-free travel experience. I did ask if all Sandals resorts catered to gluten-free needs, but they could not speak on their behalf—each destination would have to be contacted.

Bob and Ruth's Gluten-Free Dining and Travel Club, described by Mary earlier in this chapter, plans gluten-free trips all over the world, but I must admit there is one in particular that is on my dream list: the Culinary Institute of America in Hyde Park, New York. The following is a description of this tour in Bob Levy's own words:

Culinary Institute of America (CIA), [in] Hyde Park, New York, starts the evening with a wine and cheese get-together including the CIA'S Certified Master Baker Richard Coppedge. This is how the three day "glutton-gluten-free" getaway began. After a morning guided tour, and a time for shopping in the gift shop, one had a feeling of completeness having experienced the ambiance of the school setting.

Lunch was held at the Ristorante Caterina de'Medici in the magnificent Colavita Center. An afternoon wine tasting at a local organic winery, a bit of relaxation and then on to the next "glutton" experience. The elegant Escoffier Restaurant offered up a gluten-free Beef Wellington with light flaky pastry crust for this memorable dining experience.

The next day, after a full breakfast at the hotel, a tour of Eleanor Roosevelt's cottage and grounds was the first stop on the agenda. The morning was capped off with a tour of the Franklin D. Roosevelt Home and Library. Pack your bags and get ready to go on this grand excursion. There are so many great places to go and our goal is to make gluten free traveling a wonderful experience for the whole family.

Another option when traveling is to stay at a bed and breakfast (B&B). You should check with a particular B&B before you stay there. Never venture to a B&B without checking in advance to make sure they offer a gluten-free breakfast. Make sure you always do your own homework before making a reservation.

Celiac Chicks Around The World: Gluten-Free B&B in Newport, Rhode Island, was the first B&B to indicate that it had a gluten-free status. Maria wrote the following about the Celiac Chicks B&B:

I spent three days at the Architect's Inn Bed & Breakfast in Newport, RI, and aside from being owned and operated by two of the nicest, most hospitable guys around—Brian and Nick, and exquisitely decorated with Victorian antiques, I was served a fabulous gluten-free breakfast! And we're not talking just toasted "Foods by George" English muffins, oh no—try baked apples, cored and filled with dried sweetened cranberries and drizzled with maple syrup, followed by feather-light gluten-free pumpkin pancakes dusted with confectioner's sugar and topped with apple syrup (seriously, I almost cried), with a side of turkey bacon; next morning: pear parfait—pear chunks topped with Greek yogurt and honey, followed by Breakfast Risotto: risotto tossed with scrambled eggs and sautéed sugar snap peas with a side of turkey bacon (I polygamously asked Brian to marry me within earshot of my current husband).

It was heaven and if that wasn't enough, would you believe they left a plate of freshly baked gluten-free chocolate chip cookies in my room at turndown?! They also recommended an excellent allergy-sensitive restaurant in town, Tucker's Bistro, that accommodated me with a special appetizer (on New Year's Eve, no less)— and I've almost run out of adjectives here—velvety rich, perfectly seasoned butternut squash soup (all stocks are gluten-free). They also made adjustments to my other menu selections as needed, to make them gluten-free. They do vegetarian, with advance notice. And don't let me get started on the gluten-free chocolate toffee crème brûlée.

King's Cottage B&B in Lancaster, Pennsylvania, also serves a gluten-free breakfast, with advance notice. Their Web site (http://www.kingscottagebb.com) reads:

Feel yourself unwind as you travel through Lancaster County's tranquil back roads in Amish Country. Enjoy world-class entertainment, savor Pennsylvania Dutch cooking, visit historic sites, stroll art galleries, enjoy intimate gourmet restaurants—all within minutes of the King's Cottage—your home away from home. Come enjoy our wonderful Lancaster PA Bed and Breakfast.

Chicken Paradise B&B is located in San Antonio, Texas. The proprietors, Anne and Joe, have lived there since 1980, and are eager to share their San Antonio B&B oasis with others. They cater to individuals with dietary restrictions. Anne has lived a gluten-free lifestyle since she was diagnosed with CD in 1998. Their favorite kind of trip is to go to France or Italy and rent a little cottage in the country. They enjoy daily trips to visit the markets and scenes of the area and then going "home" to their little place in the evening. They are trying to offer the same idea to their guests. Your home-away-from-home accommodations at Chicken Paradise can be the Paradise Suite, a detached guest suite with private entrance available to rent by the night or by the week. Anne and Joe offer some of the same kinds of hospitality they have enjoyed over the years. A gluten-free breakfast prepared in a gluten-free environment is at the top of the list at Chicken Paradise. There is a large pool, a private outdoor (hot water) shower, a tree house, and places to read or stroll around in the serenity of the lush bed and breakfast retreat. There are chickens and peacocks roaming the premises. There also is a big organic garden, and guests are welcome to sample the herbs that grow there.

Joan, who lives gluten free, and her husband recently stayed at the Raven Haven B&B in Mentone, Alabama. Mentone is located in northeast Alabama, atop Lookout Mountain, and is close to both Georgia and Tennessee. This charming community offers all kinds of things to do, including fishing; hiking; canoeing; swimming; horseback riding; and shopping at antique galleries, gift shops, and local artisan shops. Joan was looking for relaxation, a beautiful room, and gluten-free food. Tony and Eleanor Teverino, innkeepers at Raven Haven, promised and provided all three.

The Arbor Inn B&B is located in Prescott, Wisconsin. It provides gluten-free breakfasts and offers access to many activities in the area.

The owners of Parmele House B&B, in Plattsmouth, Nebraska, invite their guests to relax in their comfortably furnished rooms, complete with rocking chairs. Antiques are blended into a Southwest decor.

I selected these B&Bs at random from different parts of the United States, to give you examples of places that cater to a gluten-free lifestyle. Do your own research and make your own list! Whether you are planning to visit Disney World, take a cruise, go camping, hike the Appalachian Trail, or go see relatives three states away requires some planning on your part to make the trip compatible with your gluten-free lifestyle. Making any venture enjoyable does take planning and a positive attitude. Even an unplanned picnic can become a gluten-free event with the right company and the right attitude.

Glossary

Acid reflux–Chronic digestive disease that occurs when stomach acid or, occasionally, bile, flows back (refluxes) into the esophagus. The backwash of acid irritates the lining of the stomach. Also known as *gastroesophageal reflux disease.*

Amaranth–Naturally gluten-free grain from the amaranth plant. Used by some food companies as a gluten-free alternative.

Anemia–Reduction in the number of red blood cells.

Antibodies–Cells the body develops when it fears it is being attacked. An antibody is a protein used by the immune system to identify and neutralize foreign objects such as bacteria and viruses. Each antibody recognizes a specific antigen unique to its target.

Aphthous stomatitis–Sores in the oral mucosa commonly called *canker sores.* Not caused by herpes simplex virus. Not uncommon in celiac disease (CD).

Arrhythmia or dysrhythmia—A disorder of the heart rate (pulse) or heart rhythm, such as beating too fast (tachycardia), too slow (bradycardia), or irregularly.

Arrowroot—An easily digested starch from the roots of the arrowroot plant.

Ataxia—Neurological symptom, occasionally seen with CD, that creates a loss of balance.

Attention-deficit/hyperactivity disorder—Condition of hyperactivity that lasts longer than three months in which the person has difficulty staying focused and being attentive.

Autoimmune disorder—A condition that occurs when the immune system mistakenly attacks and destroys healthy body tissue. There are more than eighty different types of autoimmune disorders.

Barley—A grain that has the protein hordein. It makes the body have an autoimmune response that causes CD in individuals who have a genetic predisposition.

Bean flours—Flours made from the navy, northern, pinto, lima, kidney, black, pink, garbanzo, or soy beans; black-eyed peas; or lentils. These flours are much richer in protein and fiber than traditional white flour, providing a much healthier basis for cooking in a gluten-free diet.

Buckwheat—A very nourishing, gluten-free flour that also has fiber and protein.

Carbohydrates—Come in two forms. *Simple carbohydrates* are also called *simple sugars*. Simple sugars are found in refined sugars, like the white sugar you'd find in a sugar bowl. The second form, *complex carbohydrates* are also called *starches*. Starches include grain products, such as bread, crackers, pasta, and rice. As with simple sugars, some complex carbohydrate foods are better choices than others. Refined grains, such as white flour and white rice, have been processed, which removes nutrients and fiber. But unrefined grains still contain these vitamins and minerals. Unrefined grains also are rich in fiber, which helps your digestive system work well.

Celiac disease–Medical condition in which protein from wheat, barley, and rye destroy the villi of the small intestine. Also referred to as *gluten-sensitive enteropathy, celiac sprue*, or *autoimmune enteropathy.* This is found frequently in the literature, is it not necessary to clarify?

Cerebral ataxia–Neurological condition causing disturbances of walking and balance.

Cholecystokinin–A juice secreted through a tube into the digestive tract from the pancreas. This enzyme causes the gall bladder to empty.

Choleostasis liver disease–The most common liver disorder among CD patients. Choleostasis is any condition in which the flow of bile from the liver is blocked.

Colon–Area known as the *large intestine*, which is the last part of the digestive system in most vertebrates; it extracts water and salt from solid wastes before they are eliminated from the body and is the site in which bacteria ferments the unused products not absorbed in the body.

Constipation–Inability to evacuate the lower bowel on a regular basis without the help of laxatives.

Corn–A naturally gluten-free vegetable plant. It does contain corn gluten, but that protein is not a problem for individuals who are gluten intolerant.

Crohn's disease–Inflammation of the digestive tract that most commonly affects the lower part of the small intestine called the *ilium.* The swelling extends deep into the lining of the affected area (all layers may be involved.) Also called *ileitis* or *enteritis.* Symptoms include abdominal pain, diarrhea, bloating, weight loss, and/or intestinal bleeding.

Dental enamel hypoplasia–Darkening and thinning of the teeth enamel due to lack of calcium absorption.

Depression–A serious medical illness that involves the brain. It's more than just a feeling of being "down in the dumps" or "blue" for a few days. About twenty percent of individuals with CD suffer from depression. Symptoms can include sadness; loss of interest or pleasure in activities you used to enjoy; change in weight; difficulty sleeping, or oversleeping; energy loss; feelings of worthlessness; and thoughts of death or suicide.

Dermatitis herpetiformis–A skin form of CD that creates a blistery, very itchy rash.

Diabetes mellitus–Condition in which the body has difficulty producing sufficient amounts of insulin. [Type 1 is called *insulin-dependent diabetes*. In Type 1 diabetes the body does not make insulin and therefore the blood sugar goes very high if not controlled. Type 2 diabetes, in which the body does not utilize sugar or insulin properly, is much more common and is controlled by diet and medication.

Diarrhea–Frequent loose, watery stools occurring more than normal daily.

Dietitian–A professional who specializes in food and nutrition.

Digestion–The mechanism of the body when ingesting food and the process that occurs when it is used by the body.

Down syndrome–A set of mental and physical symptoms that result from having an extra copy of chromosome 21. Even though people with Down syndrome may have some physical and mental features in common, symptoms of Down syndrome can range from mild to severe. Usually, mental development and physical development are slower in people with Down syndrome than in those without it. About twenty percent of people with Down syndrome also have CD.

Eczema–An inflammatory condition of the skin.

Endomysial antibodies–Antibodies produced by the body in reaction to the presence of the gluten in the grains of wheat, barley, or rye.

Endoscopy–Procedure that allows the gastroenterologist to examine and biopsy the esophagus, stomach, duodenum, and small intestine by using a tube (scope) with a light on it.

Enriched–When nutrients that were lost during processing are added back in.

Enteropathy–Any pathology (disease) of the intestine. Gluten sensitive enteropathy is an example.

Enzymes–Proteins that increase the rates of chemical reactions or act like a catalyst to turn them into molecules.

Esophageal sphincter–Small opening from the esophagus into the stomach that moves food into the stomach at a rate such that the stomach can start digesting.

Esophagogastroduodenoscopy–Procedure done with a gastric scope so the physician can identify the esophagus, the stomach, and the duodenum. It is used for diagnostic purposes such as CD.

Esophagus–The tube from the mouth to the stomach that carries food. It has a movement that allows the food to move slowly enough to start digestion.

Excipients–Substances used in drug products that are not the actual drug. They are fillers such as starches, coloring, or gelatin.

Extrinsic nerves–Outside nerves that come to the digestive organs from the brain or the spinal cord. They release chemicals for digestion.

Fat–Molecules that provide energy for the body and aids the body in absorbing nutrients.

Fibromyalgia–A condition that makes you feel tired and causes muscle pain and *tender points*, places on the neck, shoulders, back, hips, arms, or legs that hurt when touched. People with fibromyalgia may have other symptoms, such as trouble sleeping, morning stiffness, headaches, and problems with thinking and memory. Fibromyalgia is not uncommon in CD.

Flax–The naturally gluten-free seed of the flax plant. It is very high in fiber and should be ground to be of most value. Can be added to cereals, baked items, or casseroles.

Food Allergen Labeling and Consumer Protection Act of 2004– Mandates that eight allergens must appear on all manufacturing label of foods: (a) milk, (b) eggs, (c) fish, (d) crustacean shellfish, (e) tree nuts, (f) wheat, (g) peanuts, and (h) soybeans

Food allergy–A reaction of the immune system to something that does not bother most other people. People who have food allergies often are sensitive to more than one thing and are able to detect it if the food is avoided.

Food intolerance–A digestive system response rather than an immune system response. It occurs when something in a food irritates a person's digestive system or when a person is unable to properly digest, or break down, the food. Intolerance to lactose, which is found in milk and other dairy products, is the most common food intolerance.

Fortified–When nutrients that are not present in the original product are added

Gallbladder–A small pouch that sits just under the liver, under the right ribs. The gallbladder stores bile produced by the liver. After meals, the gallbladder is empty and flat, like a deflated balloon. Before a meal, the gallbladder may be full of bile and about the size of a small pear.

Gastrin–Hormone that causes the stomach to produce and acid for dissolving and digesting some foods.

Gastroenterologist–Physician who specializes in the gastrointestinal tract and the diagnosis, disorders, and treatment of such diseases.

Ghrelin–An enzyme produced in the stomach and upper intestine in the absence of food in the digestive system and stimulates appetite.

Gliadin–The protein that is found in wheat.

Gluten–The protein of the grain that holds a product together (e.g., bread). It comes from the Latin word meaning "glue."

Gluten-Free Certification Organization–A program launched by the Gluten Intolerance Group to determine and certify that gluten-free food products test for fewer than ten parts per million as being gluten free. Products that meet this criterion are then given the organization's label.

Gluten intolerance–Condition in which an individual becomes ill (bloated, diarrhea, gaseous) as a result of consuming any food item with gluten present. They may or may not have villi destruction as a result of this.

Gluten-sensitive enteropathy–A diagnosis frequently given in cases of CD.

Gluten sensitivity–Diagnosis reserved for individuals who have a normal biopsy and a predictable and recurring set of symptoms relieved by removing gluten from the diet.

Glutinin–One of the proteins in wheat flour.

Graves' disease–The most common cause of hyperthyroidism in the United States. Also known as toxic diffuse goiter. Hyperthyroidism is a disorder that occurs when the thyroid gland makes more thyroid hormone than the body needs.

Hashimoto's disease–A form of chronic inflammation of the thyroid gland that results in damage to the thyroid gland and reduced thyroid function or hypothyroidism, meaning the gland doesn't make enough thyroid hormone for the needs of the body. Hashimoto's disease is the most common cause of hypothyroidism in the United States. Also called *chronic lymphocytic thyroiditis* or *autoimmune thyroiditis*.

Hemoglobin–The main component of red blood cells, a protein that carries oxygen away from the lungs to the tissues.

Hepatitis–An inflammation of the liver. Hepatitis A is infectious hepatitis, hepatitis B is serum hepatitis, and hepatitis C is a viral infectious disease of the liver contacted from blood or needle contact that can result in end-stage liver disease.

Hives–Itchy raise skin rash that can caused by an allergy to food or something topical. Also know as *urticaria*.

Hordein–The protein found in barley.

Hypochondriasis–A persistent fear of having a serious medical illness. Individuals with this disorder tend to believe they have a sign of a serious disease. They may be especially concerned about a particular organ.

IgA–Immunoglobulin A, which is frequently deficient in individuals with CD.

IgE–An allergen-specific antibody test for immunoglobin E.

IgG–Immunoglobulin G, a protein in blood plasma that acts as an antibody. An IgG test can be performed if the patient has an IgA deficiency.

Indian rice grass–A plant and seed used by Native Americans. It is sold as quinoa for a gluten-free diet.

Infertility–Inability of a conjugal couple to be able to reproduce naturally within a reasonable period of time. Individuals with undiagnosed CD sometimes struggle with infertility.

Interleukin-17A–A pro-inflammatory cytokine secreted by activated T-cells. Some recent research suggests that interleukin-17A has a role in the pathogenesis of celiac disease.

Intrinsic nerves–Nerves located on the inside of the digestive tract that release substances when food is present.

Iron deficiency anemia–Condition that occurs when your blood does not carry enough oxygen to the rest of your body. The most common cause of anemia is not having enough iron. Your body needs iron to make hemoglobin. Iron deficiency anemia can be caused by blood loss, malabsorption due to damage to the intestine, or a disturbance of blood production.

Irritable bowel syndrome–A condition of the small intestine with various symptoms such as diarrhea, bloating, and abdominal pain that is not usually relieved by medication. Often misdiagnosed as CD.

Lactose intolerance–Inability of an individual to tolerate the sugar (lactose) in milk and milk products.

Legumes–Members of the bean/pea family. High in protein and gluten free.

Lentil–A bushy plant of the legume family, grown for its lens-shaped seeds, which are naturally gluten free. It is about fifteen inches (thirty-eight centimeters) tall and the seeds grow in pods, usually with two seeds in each.

Liver–Large organ located under the ribs on the right side. Its many functions include filtering blood; producing bile; converting sugar to glycogen, which it stores; and aiding in the absorption of food. It breaks down waste matter in the blood and manufacturers blood protein.

Malignancy–Cancerous growth].

Mesentery–Membrane that attaches to the body wall. Usually refers to the membrane around the small and large intestines.

Mesquite–A deeply rooted plant of the southwestern United States.

Millets–Agroup of small-seeded species of cereal crops or grains, widely grown around the world for food and fodder.

Montina–Type of flour created from milled *Indian rice grass*, a type of grass native to the western United States. Indian rice grass was grown and used by Native Americans as much as seven thousand years ago. (The grass is not related to rice.) Montina flour was determined to be gluten free by Dr. David Sands, a plant pathologist working at Montana State University.

Mucosa—The soft tissue lining of the inside of the mouth or the lining of the digestive tract.

Multiple sclerosis—Nervous system disease that affects the brain and spinal cord. It damages the myelin sheath, the material that surrounds and protects your nerve cells. This damage slows down or blocks messages between your brain and your body.

Multisystem disorder—A condition in which more than one system in the body is affected. In CD, the gastrointestinal tract is involved; however, the skin, brain, and other areas of the body also may be involved.

Myasthenia gravis—An autoimmune condition that causes the body to react to messages your nerves send to your muscles. It often affects muscles in your head. Common symptoms are trouble with eye and eyelid movement, facial expression, and swallowing.

Necrosis—Process by which an area of the body fails to get a sufficient blood supply and begins to die.

Neuropathy—Loss of nerve function to an area of the body, creating numbness or loss of feeling.

Nuts—A hard-shelled fruit of some plants and trees. All nuts can be made into flour for use in a gluten-free diet. Some are made into milk for individuals with allergies. They have protein and fiber to improve nutrients.

Oats—A naturally gluten-free grain but often is grown in areas where wheat contaminates it. For oats to be considered gluten free they should be grown separately from wheat and tested for gluten.

Osteolacia—A condition in which the bones are not receiving enough calcium. It is the first indication of calcium loss in the bones.

Osteopenia—A condition in which bone mineral density is lower than normal. It is considered by many doctors to be a precursor to osteoporosis.

Osteoporosis—Condition in which the bones have mottled openings and softness, indicating a lack of calcium and high risk of fracture.

Pancreas—Gland that secretes insulin and pancreatic juice to assist digestion in the small intestine.

Peptide YY—Enzyme produced in the digestive tract in response to a meal in the system and inhibits appetite.

Peripheral neuropathy—Damage to nerve endings, causing a loss of feeling in the fingers, toes, or other body parts.

Potato flour—A very white starch powder, made from potatoes, used as a thickening agent. Often confused with potato starch. It is a peeled, cooked potato which has been mashed, dried, and ground, that includes the fiber and protein.

Potato starch—Very white starch powder used as a thickening agemt. Is obtained by grinding the tubers to a pulp and removing the fiber and protein by water-washings.. Not the same thing as potato flour.

Prolamins—A group of plant storage proteins having a high proline content and found in the seeds of cereal grains such as wheat (gliadin).

Proteins—Polymer chains made of amino acids linked together by peptide bonds. Amino acids can be divided into either *essential amino acids* or *nonessential amino acids*. Proteins are found in every living cell in the body. Our bodies need protein from the foods we eat to build and maintain bones, muscles, and skin. We get proteins in our diet from meat, dairy products, nuts, and certain grains and beans.

Refractory celiac disease—Persistent or recurrent malabsorptive symptoms and villous atrophy despite strict adherence to a gluten-free diet for at least six to twelve months in the absence of other causes of nonresponsive celiac disease.

Rice—A cereal grain, the most important staple food for a large part of the world's human population, especially in eastern and southern Asia, the Middle East, Latin America, and the West Indies. It is the grain with the second-highest worldwide production, after corn.

Rye—Grain with the protein secalin that produces CD in individuals who have a genetic predisposition.

Salivary glands—Glands under the oral cavity that secrete liquid for beginning digestion in the mouth.

Secalin—The protein found in rye.

Secretin—Enzyme that causes the pancreas to send out a digestive juice that is rich in bicarbonate. It helps neutralize the acidic stomach contents as they enter the small intestine.

Sepsis—Poisoning of the system by disease-producing bacteria and their toxins, which are absorbed into the bloodstream.

Sjögren's syndrome—Autoimmune disease that occurs in middle-aged or older women. Symptoms include dryness of the mouth, inflammation of the eyes, and enlargement of the parotid glands, the small glands that produce saliva into the mouth.

Small intestine—The part of the digestive tract that extends from the stomach to the large intestine. This area digests most of the food and distributes the nourishment where it is needed. It is the area that has the villi that are destroyed by the proteins in wheat, barley, and rye in CD.

Sorghum—Plant that can be made into flour that is gluten free.

Soy—Plant that is high in protein, can be made into flour, and is gluten free.

Sprue—A name that previously was used to identify CD (*celiac sprue*). It was probably derived from the Dutch word *sprew*.

Stomach–The part of the digestive tract that goes from the esophagus to the small intestine. It secretes digestive enzymes to begin breaking up food particles.

Systemic lupus erythematosis–Condition in which the immune system attacks healthy cells and tissues by mistake. This can damage the joints, skin, blood vessels and organs.

Tapioca–The root of the cassava plant that can be made into a white starch used for thickening and puddings. It is naturally gluten free.

T-cell lymphoma–A non-Hodgkins type of cancer that is usually caused by the autoimmune system reacting to the body's continued exposure to an environmental-causing inflammatory process (e.g., wheat, barley, or rye) in genetically susceptible individuals There are many types of T-cell lymphoma, including enteropathy T-cell lymphoma, an extremely rare subtype that appears in the intestines and is strongly associated with CD.

Teff–A cereal plant used mainly in Ethiopia. It is naturally gluten free.

Tissue transglutaminase (tTG)–The enzyme that is present when one has CD. tTG2 is the enzyme found in the gut of a person with CD, tTG3 is the enzyme present when the skin is biopsied at the site of dermatitis herpetiformis, and tTG6 is the enzyme found in the nervous system of CD patients with neurological disorders.

Turner syndrome–A genetic disorder whereby one X chromosome is missing, which produces short stature and loss of ovarian function. It occurs only in females.

Ulcerative colitis–Inflammation and sores in the lining of the rectum and colon. Symptoms include diarrhea, abdominal pain, anemia, fatigue, loss of appetite, weight loss, rectal bleeding, skin lesions, joint pain, and growth failure (in children).

U.S. Food and Drug Administration–A government organization with the authority to approve all drug products produced for legal use in the United States. It requires the manufacturer (pharmaceutical company) to meet many standards before a drug is approved for distribution.

Villi–Small fingerlike projections in the small intestine that absorb the nutrients of the food that one eats.

Villous atrophy–Damage to the villi of the small intestine.

Wheat–A grain that has the protein gliadin. This creates CD in individuals who have a genetic predisposition.

Wild rice–A plant grown in North American waters, very rich in protein, used for food. It is gluten free.

Williams syndrome–A condition that presents with growth delays both before and after birth and involves varying mental deficiencies. Characteristics include a round face, full cheeks, thick lips, large mouth (usually open), broad nasal bridge, flared eyebrows, small lower jaw, and prominent ears. Individuals with this condition have an awkward gait, poor motor skills, and a short attention span. Also called *Williams Beuren syndrome*.

Xanthun gum–Substance added to gluten-free baked products to add elasticity to the dough.

Zonulin–An enzyme found in the small intestine that affects the permeability of the small intestine. It is being researched as a product that might assist individuals with CD to be able to ingest it before a meal and prevent the autoimmune response.

Resources

Medical Centers With Research Areas for Celiac Research

University of Maryland School of Medicine
Center for Celiac Research
20 Penn Street, Room S303B
Baltimore, MD 21201
Appointment Lines: 410-328-6749 or 800-492-5538
Web site: http://medschool.umaryland.edu/celiac
Contact: Pam King, Director of Operations (pking@peds.
  umaryland.edu)

Celiac Clinic, University of Maryland Medical Center
22 S. Greene Street (N5W40)
Baltimore, MD 21201

The Celiac Center at Beth Israel Deaconess Medical Center
East Campus, Dana 601
330 Brookline Avenue
Boston, MA 02215
Phone: 617-667-1272
Web site: http://bidmc.org

Celiac Disease Research Program and Celiac Disease Clinic
Division of Gastroenterology and Hepatology
Mayo Clinic
200 First Street SW
Rochester, MN 55905
Phone: 507-284-2511
Web site: www.mayoclinic.com

University of Virginia Digestive Health Center of Excellence
1215 Lee Street
Charlottesville, VA 22908
Phone: 800-251-3627
Web site: www.hsc.virginia.edu

Celiac Disease Center at Columbia University
Harkness Pavilion
180 Fort Washington Avenue, Suite 934
New York, NY 10032
Phone: 212-342-4529
Fax: 212-342-0447
E-mail: celiac@columbia.edu
Web site: www.celiacdiseasecenter.org

The Center for Celiac Disease at The Children's Hospital of
    Philadelphia
34th Street and Civic Center Boulevard
Philadelphia, PA 19104
Phone: 215-590-1000

Physician Referral Service: 800-879-2467
Web site: www.chop.edu/service/center-for-celiac-disease/home.
   html

Adult Celiac Disease Program Rush University
   Medical Center
Section of Gastroenterology & Nutrition
1725 W. Harrison, Suite 207
Chicago, IL 60612
Phone: 312-942-8570
Web site: www.rush.edu/rumc/page-1175113041252.html

University of Chicago Celiac Disease Center
5839 S. Maryland Ave., MC 4065
Chicago, IL 60637
Phone: 773-702-7593
E-mail: info@celiacdisease.net
Web site: www.celiacdisease.net

Celiac Disease Clinic at the University of Colorado, Denver
Phone: 800-621-7621
Web site: www.uch.edu

Celiac Disease Clinic and Inflammatory Bowel
   Disease Center
Carver College of Medicine, University of Iowa, Iowa City
Web site: www.uihealthcare.com

Pediatric Celiac Center, Englewood Hospital and
   Medical Center
350 Engle Street
Englewood, NJ 07631
Phone: 201-894-3690.
Web site: www.englewoodhospital.com/Pediatrics/
   Pediatric_celiac_center.htm

William K. Warren Medical Research Center for Celiac Disease
University of California San Diego
9500 Gilman Drive
La Jolla, CA 92093-0623
Phone: 858-822-1022
E-mail: celiaccenter@ucsd.edu
Web site: www.celiaccenter.ucsd.edu

Celiac Center at Children's Hospital Los Angeles
Phone: 323-361-2181
Web site: www.childrenshospitalla.org
Stanford University Medical Center Celiac Sprue Clinic
Phone: 650-723-6961
Web site: www.stanfordhospital.org

Celiac Disease Program at Children's National Medical Center
111 Michigan Avenue Washington, DC 20010
Phone: 202-476-3032
Web site: www.childrensnational.org

Books

Blumer, I., and Crowe, S. (2010). *Celiac disease for dummies*. New York: John Wiley and Sons.

Bower, S. L., Sharrett, M. K., and Plogsted, S. (2006). *Celiac disease: A guide to living with gluten intolerance* . New York: Demos Health Publishing.

Brown, M. (2009). *Gluten-free, hassle free: A simple, sane, dietitian-approved program for eating your way back to health*. New York: Demos Health Publishing.

Case, S. (2010). *Gluten-free diet: A comprehensive resource guide— Expanded and revised edition*. Regina, Saskatchewan, Canada: Case Nutrition Consulting.

Crangle, C. (2002). *Living well with celiac disease: Abundance beyond wheat or gluten*. Victoria, British Columbia, Canada: Trafford.

Dowler Shepard, J. E. (2008). *The first year: Celiac disease and living gluten-free: An essential guide for the newly diagnosed.* Cambridge, MA: DaCapo Press.

Gallagher, E. (2009). *Gluten-free food science and technology.* Chichester, United Kingdom: Wiley Blackwell.

Green, P. H. R., and Jones, R. (2006).(2010) *Celiac disease: A hidden epidemic.* New York: William Morrow.

Holt, S. (2009). *Eat well live well with gluten intolerance: Gluten-free recipes and tips.* New York: Sky Horse.

Korn, D. (2001). *Kids with celiac disease: A family guide to raising happy, healthy, gluten-free children.* Bethesda, MD: Woodbine House.

Korn, D. (2006). *Living gluten-free for dummies.* New York: John Wiley and Sons.

Lieberman, S. (2006). *The gluten connection: How gluten sensitivity may be sabotaging your health—And what you can do to take control now.* New York: Rodale Books.

Petersen, V., and Petersen, R. (2009). *The gluten effect: How "innocent" wheat is ruining your health.* Hueytown, AL: True Health.

Ries, L. (2003). *What? No wheat? A lighthearted primer to living the gluten-free wheat-free life* . Phoenix, AZ: What? No Wheat? Enterprises.

Thompson, T. (2008). *The gluten-free nutrition guide.* New York: McGraw-Hill.

Wangen, S. (2009). *Healthier without wheat: A new understanding of wheat allergies, celiac disease, and non-celiac gluten intolerance.* Seattle, WA: Innate Health Publishing.

Willingham, T. (2000). *Food allergy field guide: A lifestyle manual for families.* Littleton, CO: Savory Palate.

Cookbooks

Fenster, C. (2007). *Gluten-free quick & easy: From prep to plate without the fuss—200+ recipes for people with food sensitivities.* London: Penguin.

Fenster, C. (2008). *1,000 gluten-free recipes*. Hoboken, NJ: Wiley.

Fenster, C. (2010). *100 best gluten-free recipes*. Hoboken, NJ: Wiley.

Hagman, B. (1999). *The gluten-free gourmet bakes bread: More than 200 wheat-free recipes*. New York: Henry Holt.

Hagman, B. (2000). *The gluten-free gourmet cooks fast and healthy: Wheat and gluten free with less fuss and less fat*. New York: Henry Holt.

Hagman, B. (2000). *The gluten-free gourmet: Living well without wheat*. 2nd ed. New York: Henry Holt.

Hagman, B. (2000). *More from the gluten-free gourmet: Delicious dining without wheat*. New York: Henry Holt.

Hagman, B. (2002). *The gluten-free gourmet makes dessert*. New York: Henry Holt.

Hagman, B. (2004). *The gluten-free gourmet cooks comfort foods: Creating old favorites with the new flours*. New York: Henry Holt.

Lord, S. (2009). *Getting your kid on a gluten-free casein-free diet*. London: Jessica Kingsley.

Reilly, R. (2002). *Gluten-free baking: More than 125 recipes for delectable sweet and savory baked goods, including cakes, pies, quick breads, muffins, cookies, and other delights*. New York: Simon & Schuster.

Roberts, A. G., and Pillow, C. (2010). *The gluten-free good health cookbook: The delicious way to strengthen your immune system and neutralize inflammation* Evanston, IL: Agate.

Ryberg, R. (2000). *The gluten-free kitchen: Over 135 delicious recipes for people with gluten intolerance or wheat allergy*. Roseville, CA: Prima.

Sanderson, S. L. (2002). *Incredible edible gluten-free food for kids*. Bethesda, MD: Woodbine House.

Sarros, C. (2004). *Wheat-free, gluten-free cookbook for kids and busy adults*. 2nd ed. New York: McGraw-Hill.

Sarros, C. (2004). *The wheat-free gluten-free dessert cookbook: Cooking gluten free* . New York: McGraw-Hill.

Magazines

Gluten Intolerance Group Magazine (published quarterly; included in membership)www.gluten.net
Gluten-Free Living
www.glutenfreeliving.com
Living Without
www.livingwithout.com
Scott Free Newsletter
www.celiac.com

Shopping Guides

● Clan Thompson
  Shopping guide database for a PC and Palm OS
  Pocket shopping guide
  www.clanthompson.com

● Bob and Ruth's Dining and Travel Club
  www.bobandruths.com

● Tri-County Celiac Support Group Shopping Guide and Newsletter
  www.tccsg.com

Internet Opportunities

● listserv.icors.org/archives/celiac.html
  Celiac Discussion List archives, a listserv with several thousand members who write daily about problems and questions regarding celiac disease. Answers are provided by other people who live with celiac disease. Few professionals are involved.

● www.celiackids.com
  The site for Raising Our Celiac Kids

● www.celiac.com
  Site contains very good general information, recipes, and research.

- www.gfrestaurants.com
- www.glutenfreeregistry.com
  A resource that lists restaurants by geographic location.
- www.glutenfreetravelsites.com/restaurants

General Information

- American Celiac Disease Alliance: www.americanceliac.org
- Center for Celiac Research: www.celiaccenter.org
- Gluten Freeda: www.glutenfreeda.com
- National Digestive Diseases Information Clearinghouse: www. digestive.niddk.nih.gov
- National Institute of Health Consensus Conference on Celiac Disease: http://consensus.nih.gov/2004/2004CeliacDisease11 8main.htm
- Steve Plogstedt, PharmD, medication list: www.gluten-freedrugs.com
- University of Chicago: www.uchospitals.edu/specialties
- U.S. Dry Bean Council: www.beansforhealth.org
- U.S. Department of Agribusiness: www.mypyramid.org

National Support and Resource Groups

Canadian Celiac Association
Phone: 905-507-6208
Web site: www.celiac.ca

Celiac Disease Foundation
13251 Ventura Boulevard, Suite 1
Studio City, CA 91604
Phone: 818-990-2354
Web site: www.celiac.org

Celiac Sprue Association, United States of America
Phone: 402-558-0600
Web site: www.csaceliacs.org

Gluten Intolerance Group of North America (GIG)
Phone: 253-833-6655
Web site: www.gluten.net

GIG has support groups throughout the United States. It publishes a quarterly magazine that keeps up with all of the most recent research on celiac disease. It has tremendous resources to assist its support groups. The following programs are part of the GIG organization:

Gluten-Free Certification Program: www.gfco.org

Gluten-Free Restaurant Awareness Program: www.glutenfreerestaurants.org

Gluten-Free Food Service Accreditation Program

National Foundation for Celiac Awareness
P.O. Box 544
Ambler, PA 19002
Web site: www.celiaccentral.org

Vendors of Gluten-Free Products

Fourteen years ago it was possible to count the number of gluten-free vendors on the fingers of one hand. Now there are so many that it would be impossible to include them all in this book. The more familiar you get with purchasing gluten-free food, the easier it will be to identify the vendors who produce only gluten-free items and differentiate those you like and dislike. General Mills has become a player in the field, which means more of the larger food manufacturers will get involved. Most health food stores still carry the largest variety of gluten-free foods, but the mainline grocery stores are now getting interested in carrying products and making their own gluten-free sections for your convenience. This will certainly help people who are living a gluten-free lifestyle. Many vendors market their products only over the Internet. This is very convenient for families that live in rural areas with no health food stores or large grocery stores nearby.

1-2-3 Gluten Free: www.123glutenfree.com

Amazing Grains: www.amazinggrains.com

Amy's Kitchen: www.amyskitchen.com

Authentic Foods: www.authenticfoods.com

Bob's Red Mill Natural Foods: www.bobsredmill.com

Chebe Bread: www.chebe.com

Cecelia's Marketplace: www.ceceliasmarketplace.com

Econatural Solutions/The Ruby Range: www.therubyrange.com

Edwards and Sons Trading Company: www.edwardsandsons.
com

El Peto Products: www.elpeto.com

Ener-G Foods: www.ener-g.com

Enjoy Life Foods: www.enjoylifefoods.com

Food For Life Baking Company: www.food-for-life.com

Garden Spot Distributors: www.gardenspotdist.com

Gifts of Nature: www.giftsofnature.com

Gluten-Free Meals: www.gfmeals.com

The Gluten-Free Mall: www.glutenfreemall.com

Gluten-Free Pantry: www.glutenfree.com

The Gluten-Free Trading Company: www.glutenfree.net

Gluten Solutions: www.glutensolutions.com

Healthy Chef Creations: www.healthychefcreations.com

Kingsmill Foods: www.kingsmillfoods.com

Kinnikinnick Foods: www.kinnikinnick.com

Manna From Anna: www.glutenrevolution.com

Maple Grove Foods: www.maplegrovefoods.com

Masuya: www.masuyanaturally.com

Mrs. Leepers: www.mrsleepers.com

Nature's Path: www.naturespath.com

Nu-World: www.nuworldfoods.com

Organic Valley Products www.organicvalley.coop/products/
gluten-free-products

Pamela's Products www.pamelasproducts.com

Purfoods Gluten Free www.purfoodsfreshstart.com

Rizopia Food Products, Inc. ww.rizopia.com

Silly Yak Bakery www.freshglutenfree.net
Sylvan Border Farms www.sylvanborders.com
Tinkyada www.tinkyada.com
Udis Gluten Free Foods www.udisglutenfree.com
Vans International Foods www.vanswaffles.com

504 Plan Roadmap for the Accommodation of a Student with Celiac Disease

A resource created by the National Foundation fro Celiac Awareness (NFCA)

This roadmap is not meant to be legal advice nor definitive resource. Rather, it is insight into this process and should be adjusted for individual circumstances.

Section 504 is part of the Rehabilitation Act of 1973, and applies to all institutions receiving federal financial assistance, such as public schools. Under this law, public schools must provide a free appropriate public education and not discriminate against disabled students.

This law acknowledges that the disability may not require special education services but a plan is needed to ensure the student receives an appropriate education accommodating the disability within the classroom. This law must accommodate a special diet, including a gluten-free diet, the only known treatment for celiac disease.

STUDENT INFORMATION

- Name of the Student
- Name of Student's Parents
- Date of Birth of the Student
- Grade of the Student
- School Child Attends
- Name of the School District
- Date of the Current 504 Meeting
- Date of the Next 504 Meeting

504 TEAM INFORMATION

- Child's Parents and contact information
- Primary Classroom Teacher
- School Nurse
- 504 Coordinator
- School Counselor or Psychologist
- Director of Foodservices or Cafeteria

BACKGROUND INFORMATION

What is celiac disease?

Celiac disease is a hereditary autoimmune disease that damages the villi of the small intestine and interferes with absorption of nutrients from food. What does this mean? Put simply, the body is attacking itself! Celiac disease is triggered by consumption of the protein called gluten, which is found in wheat, barley and rye. When people with celiac disease eat foods containing gluten, their immune system responds by damaging the fingerlike villi of the small intestine. When the villi become damaged, the body is unable to absorb nutrients into the bloodstream.

National Foundation for Celiac Awareness |P.O. Box 544, Ambler, PA 19002
215!325!1306 | www.CeliacCentral.org | info@celiaccentral.org

What is the treatment?

The only treatment for celiac disease is a 100%, life-long gluten-free diet, which means avoiding all forms of wheat, barley and rye. A special caution must be given to oats, which in their natural form do not contain the gluten protein. However, most fields where oats are grown and mills that produce and store oats also manufacture wheat, barley or rye, resulting in cross-contamination. Current research shows that the majority of patients with celiac disease can tolerate oats in their pure, uncontaminated form. It is important that oat consumption be limited to oats with one of the following labels: "pure, uncontaminated oats, " "gluten-free, " or "certified gluten-free oats." It is recommended that oats be introduced under medical supervision and slowly.

Despite these restrictions, people with celiac disease can eat a well-balanced diet that consists of healthy and delicious foods. Even though it may seem impossible to maintain the diet at school, these simple guidelines will ensure that your child has the best possible experience throughout their school years.

OVERVIEW OF THE CHILD'S CONDITION
- History of celiac disease of child:
  - o Year of diagnosis
  - o Amount of time on a gluten-free diet

- Basis for the determination of the disability:
  - o Refer to letter from doctor/physician initiating 504 plan

- Disability that affects a major life activity:
  - o Restricted diet, gluten-free

- Child's developmental level and needs:
  - o Self-reliance for the student in managing their diet and disease. This fluctuates individually and developmentally. Some indicators of a child's readiness: The student is always able to visually recognize the allergen in all its hidden forms or part of another food (starch, malt, play dough, etc.).
    _____Yes _____No
  - o The student is always able to read labels for gluten.
    _____Yes _____No
  - o The student is always able to verbally communicate body discomfort associated with a reaction. _____Yes _____No
  - o The student always knows to wash his/her hands well with an approved soap and warm water before eating. _____Yes _____No

  - o The student always knows to eat only food brought from home. (If arranged)
    _____Yes _____No

National Foundation for Celiac Awareness |P.O. Box 544, Ambler, PA 19002
215!32!1306 | www.CeliacCentral.org | info@celiaccentral.org

o The student always knows not to trade food wi th classmates and adults.
_____Yes _____No

o The student always understands h ow a safe food may become cross-contaminated with gluten. _____Yes _____No

GOALS OF THE 504 PLAN - examples
1. Adhering to all aspects of the 504 Plan to avoid gluten.
2. Assisting the child to maintain a stable physiological state void of gluten reactions through preventative measures.
3. Recognizing the signs of a reaction and treating it promptly in all school contexts.
4. Striking a balance between safety and social normalcy, providing the same opportunities and conditions as the child's peers, and offering encouragement to the child.
5. Encouraging open and on-going communication among adults about food intolerance issues and doing so discretely and in the appropriate forum.

PART F: FOOD ALLERGY EDUCATION, AWARENESS & REACTION PREVENTION
The basic question to be answered and discussed in this section: What kind of training needs to take place to promote education, awareness and reaction prevention in the school context?
Types of Education, Awareness and Reaction Prevention:
- Label reading.
- Proper hand washing.
- What is cross contamination and how can it be avoided?
- Effective table and desk washing with appropriate chemicals and materials
- Positive role modeling (Example: A positive role model would not make statements to parents and students such as, "We cannot have a holiday party because of "Suzy" Celiac and her food allergies." A positive role model would say, "We are going to ha ve a holiday party and we will make it fun and safe for everyone.")
- Promotion of positive self-esteem for child with celiac disease .
- Promotion of peer support for child with celiac disease.

COMMUNICATION MANAGEMENT
A plan should be made for communication amongst those on the team and possibly include a provision for parents to be included in all communication about this subject. The most important conduits in the communication management plan will between the parents and the school cafeteria or food provider and the parents and the homeroom or primary teacher. A communication plan should be available in the event a substitute is covering a class.

CLASSROOM MANAGEMENT
- Parent and teacher will work together to mo nitor classroom events that may include the use of food.
- An alternative to using food treats for students' birthdays can be selected.
- Class activities using envelopes will be minimized and child reminded not to lick any envelope/stickers in class.

- Student should be allowed bathroom privileges when necessary.
- Student must be careful with use of the following materials for classroom projects or completely avoid their use: play dough, paper mache, fruit loops and cheerios and other gluten containing food, pasta, flour, paste, envelope and stamp adhesives. Hands and surfaces must be completely washed after the use of these materials. Parents will provide a list of alternative materials if the class plans to use any of these materials.
- The teacher will communicate with parents about upcoming projects that may require alternative foods or materials.

Nurse or Medical Department
- Faculty and staff training regarding the plan.
- Provide presentation and or information to staff and class on celiac disease and the gluten-free diet.

Art Room
- Food will not be distributed in the art classroom.
- Products commonly used in the art room will be reviewed to determine that they are gluten-free. Any changes in art products will be communicated prior to instituting the change. (e.g. paper mache and play dough)
- Student must be careful with use of the following materials for classroom projects or completely avoid their use: play dough, paper mache, fruit loops and cheerios and other gluten containing food, pasta, flour, paste, envelope and stamp adhesives. Hands and surfaces must be completely washed after the use of these materials. Parents will provide a list of alternative materials if the class plans to use any of these materials.

Food Services
- Food handling procedures that introduce gluten-free foods and prevent cross contamination are essential. The National Foundation for Celiac Awareness has a training program in place for schools called GREAT Schools. More information can be found by visiting: www.CeliacLearning.com.
- Assimilation: A goal of this is to assimilate the child into the regular structures of the school.
- Separate is often unequal and kitchens are encouraged to have students on a gluten-free diet have the same choices as other students, just gluten-free
- It is the parent's responsibility to review food and approve items
- The kitchen then is responsible to appraise parent of changes
- Some options tried by other schools:
    o All side items are gluten-free
    o One day a week one entrée is gluten-free but available for everyone.
    o Bring in quick items to substitute: hamburger buns or pizza crust.
- Parent and Food Services will work together to arrange procedures when student is ordering school lunch or bringing food from home that will require heating in the cafeteria. (e.g. warming in the oven on a separate foiled cookie sheet).

National Foundation for Celiac Awareness |P.O. Box 544, Ambler, PA 19002
215!325!1306 | www.CeliacCentral.org | info@celiaccentral.org

Field Trips
- Teachers will communicate to parent if food will be provided as part of field trip. Parent will determine whether food is gluten-free and/or provide student with a safe alternative. Parents will have the option of keeping a child home if no provisions can be made without penalty to the student.

Some other topics to be considered in this section:
- Safety snack box provided by the family to be kept in classroom
- Birthdays
- After school events such as pizza night consider utilizing one of the many companies now providing gluten-free options: Zpizza, Godfather's Pizza, Garlic Jims.
- Holiday parties
- In case of reaction: access to bathroom.
- Emergency kits: If your school has kits for emergencies or evacuation, then what supplies will be provided for those on a gluten-free diet and by whom?

National Foundation for Celiac Awareness |P.O. Box 544, Ambler, PA 19002
215!325!1306 | www.CeliacCentral.org | info@celiaccentral.org

Bibliography

Chapter 1

Accomando S., Cataldo F. (2004). The global village of celiac disease. *Digestive and liver disease: official journal of the Italian Society of Gastroenterology and the Italian Association for the Study of the Liver* 36(7):492-8.

Adams, A. (2010). Symptoms of gluten allergy. *Gluten Intolerance Group Magazine,* (33): 1, 2, 4.

Ciacca, C., Iavarone, A., Siniscalchi, M., Romano, R., and DeRosa, A. (2002). Psychological dimensions of celiac disease: Toward an integrative approach. *Digestive Diseases and Sciences* 47:2082-7.

Fasano, A. (2009). Surprises from celiac disease *Scientific American* 301(2): 54-61.

Green, P. (2010). Cutting through the confusion. *Gluten-Free Living*, No. 2, pp. 28-29, 44.

Haynes, A. J., and Savill, A. (2008). *The food intolerance bible.* San Francisco: Conan Press.

Nelsen, D. A. (2002). Gluten-sensitive enteropathy (celiac disease): More common than you think. *American Family Physician* 66:2259-66.

Pinto Sánchez, M. I., Smecuol, E., Vázquez, H., Mazure, R., et al. (2009). Very high rate of misdiagnosis of celiac disease in clinical practice. *Acta Gastroenterologica Latinoamericana* 39:250-3.

Sapone, A., Lammers, K. M., Mazzarella, G., Mikhailenko, I., et al. (2010). Differential mucosal IL-17 expression in two gliadin-induced disorders: Gluten sensitivity and the autoimmune enteropathy celiac disease. *International Archives of Allergy and Immunology* 152:75-80.

Sicherer, S. H. (2006). *Understanding and managing your child's food allergies*. Baltimore: Johns Hopkins University Press.

Silberberg, B. (2009). *The autism and ADHD diet*. Naperville, IL: Sourcebooks.

Tack, G. J., Verbeek, W. H., Schreurs, M. W., and Mulder, C. J. (2010). The spectrum of celiac disease: Epidemiology, clinical aspects and treatment. *Nature Reviews: Gastroenterology and Hepatology* 7:204-13.

Whalen, A. (2010). *Using diet to treat autism. Gluten-Free Living*, No. X, pp. 40-42.

Chapter 2

Gasbarrini, G., Miele, L., Corazza, G. R., and Gasbarrini, A. (2010). When was celiac disease born? The Italian case from the archeologic site of Cosa. *Journal of Clinical Gastroenterology* 44:502-3.

Guandalini, S. (2007). History of celiac disease. *Impact Magazine*, Summer, p. 1.

Losowsky, M. S. (2008). A history of ceoliac disease. *Digestive Diseases* 26:112-20.

Ratner, A. (2010). Dr. Allesio Fasano on the future of celiac disease. *Gluten-Free Living*, No. 4, pp. 41-42, 48.

Stone, D. (2010, April). *National Celiac Awareness Month and history of celiac disease*. http://www.celiac.com/articles/22076/1/

National-Celiac-Awareness-Month-and-History-of-Celiac-Disease/Page1.html (accessed December 26, 2010).

Walker, M. M., and Murray, J. A. (2010, November 3). An update in the diagnosis of ceoliac disease. *Histopathology.* Epub ahead of print. doi:10.1111/j.1365-2559.2010.03680.x

Chapter 3

Abenavoli, L. (2010). Brain hypoperfusion and neurological symptoms in celiac disease. *Movement Disorders* 25:792-3.

Adams, A. L. (2010). The sensitivity and specificity of celiac disease blood tests. *Gluten Intolerance Group Magazine* 32(4): 1-2, 4, 5.

Bahari, A., Karimi, M., Sanei-Moghaddam, I., Firouzi, F., and Hashemi, M. (2010). Prevalence of celiac disease among blood donors in Sistan and Balouchestan Province, southeastern Iran. *Archives of Iranian Medicine* 13:301-5.

Biagi, F., and Corazza, G. R. (2010). Mortality in celiac disease. *Nature Reviews: Gastroenterology and Hepatology* 7:158-62.

Differences in celiac disease, gluten intolerance and gluten sensitivity. (2009). *Gluten Intolerance Group Education Bulletin,* April.

Egan, L. J., Stevens, F. M., and McCarthy, C. F. (1996). Celiac disease and T-cell lymphoma. *New England Journal of Medicine* 335:1611-12.

Freeman, H. J. (2010). Mesenteric lymph node cavitation syndrome. *World Journal of Gastroenterology* 16(24): 2991-3.

Green, P. (2010, February). Cutting through the confusion. *Gluten-Free Living,* No. 2, pp. 28-29, 44.

Hadjivassiliou, M., Sanders, D. S., Grünewald, R, A., Woodroofe, N., et al. (2010). Gluten sensitivity: From gut to brain. *The Lancet Neurology* 9:318-30.

Häuser, W., Janke, K. H., Klump, B., Gregor, M., and Hinz, A. (2010). Anxiety and depression in adult patients with celiac disease on a gluten-free diet. *World Journal of Gastroenterology* 16: 2780-7.

Kurppa, K., Ashorn, M., Iltanen, S., Koskinen, L. L., et al. (2010). Celiac disease without villous atrophy in children: A prospective study. *Journal of Pediatrics* 157:373-80.

Rubio-Tapia, A., Rahim, M. W., See, J. A., Lahr, B. D., et al. (2010). Mucosal recovery and mortality in adults with celiac disease after treatment with a gluten-free diet. *American Journal of Gastroenterology* 105:1412-20.

Sapone, A., Lammers, K. M., Mazzarela, G., Mikhailenko, I., et al. (2010). Differential mucosal IL-17 expression in two gliadin-induced disorders: Gluten sensitivity and the autoimmune enteropathy celiac disease. *International Archives of Allergy and Immunology* 152:75-80.

Sieniawski, M., Angamuthu, N., Boyd, K., Chasty, R., et al. (2010). Evaluation of enteropathy associated T-cell lymphoma comparing standard therapies with a novel regimen including autologous stem cell transplantation. *Blood* 115:3664-70.

Sollid, L. M. (2002). Coeliac disease: Dissecting a complex disorder. *Nature Reviews: Immunology* 2:647-55.

Terasaki, G. S., and Ajam, K. S. (2009). Revisiting celiac disease. *Postgraduate Medicine* 121:166-9.

Tontini, G. E., Rondonotti, E., Saladino, V., Saibeni, S., et al. (2010). Impact of gluten withdrawal on health-related quality of life in celiac subjects: An observational case-control study. *Digestion* 82:221-8.

Chapter 4

Digestive system and how it functions (n.d.). http://digestive.niddk.nih.gov/diseases (accessed November 15, 2010).

Chapter 5

Sharrett, M. K. (2004, November). Gluten-free ways to increase fiber intake. Unpublished conference handout.

Chapter 6

Ciacca, C., Iavarone, A., Siniscalchi, M., Romano, R., and DeRosa, A. (2002). Psychological dimensions of celiac disease: Toward an integrative approach. *Digestive Diseases and Sciences* 47:2082-7.

DeRosa, A., Troncone, A., Vacca, M., and Ciacci, C. (2004). Characteristics and quality of illness behavior in celiac disease. *Psychosomatics* 45:336-42.

USA Today. (2010, May). [Sixteen page supplement on celiac disease sponsored by gluten-free vendors.]

Chapter 7

Kupper, C. (2010, Spring). ADA's guidelines help dietitians help you. *Gluten Intolerance Group Magazine*, pp. 18, 23, 48.

Chapter 8

Alcohol in the gluten-free diet: Quick start diet guide for celiac disease. (2010). *Gluten Intolerance Group Education Bulletin*, August.

Egan, K. (2010). Interview with Richard Coppedge. *Gluten-Free Living*, No. 2, pp. 38-39, 48.

Coppedge, R. (2008). *Gluten-free baking with the Culinary Institute of America.* Avon, MA: Adams Media.

Fenster, C. (2008). *1,000 gluten-free recipes.* Hoboken, NJ: Wiley.

Fenster, C. (2010). Can this sponge make me sick? Food safety in the kitchen. *Gluten-Free Living*, No. 1, pp. 20-21, 24, 25.

Jankowiak, C., and Ludwig, D. (2008). Frequent causes of diarrhea: Celiac disease and lactose intolerance *Medizinische Klinik* 103:413-22.

Chapter 9

Carassi, C., and Fasano, A. (2010). Celiac disease diagnosis: Simple rules are better than complicated algorithms. *American Journal of Medicine* 123:691-3.

Dorn, S. D., Hernandez, L., Minaya, M. T., Morris, C. B., et al. (2010). Psychosocial factors are more important than disease activity in determining gastrointestinal symptoms and health status in adults at a celiac disease referral center. *Digestive Diseases and Sciences* 55:3154-63.

Holmes, S. (2010). Coeliac disease: Symptoms, complications and patient support. *Nursing Standard* 24(35):50-6.

Jankowiak, C., and Ludwig, D. (2008). Frequent causes of diarrhea: Celiac disease and lactose intolerance *Medizinische Klinik* 103:413-22.

Kohnle, D. (2010, August 13). *Signs that you may have celiac disease.* HealthDay News. http://www.mentalhelp.net/poc/view_doc.php?type=news&id=130631&cn=281 (accessed January 7, 2011).

Rodrigo-Sáez, L., and Pérez-Martínez, I. (2010). Adult celiac disease—A common, significant health problem worldwide. *Revista Española de Enfermedades Digestivas* 102:461-5.

Rubio-Tapia, A., Barton, S. H., and Murray, J. A. (2011). Celiac disease and persistent symptoms. *Clinical Gastroenterology and Hepatology* 9:13-17.

Rubio-Tapia, A., and Murray, J. (2010). Classification and management of refractory celiac disease. *Gut* 59:547-57.

Update on celiac disease: New standards and new tests. (2010, Summer). *Gluten Intolerance Group Magazine*, p. 15.

Wang, X. Q., Liu, W., Xu, J. J., Mei, H., et al. (2010). Prevalence of celiac disease in children with chronic diarrhea in China. *Chinese Journal of Pediatrics* 48:244-8.

Chapter 10

Blumer, I., and Crowe, S. (2010). *Celiac disease for dummies.* New York: John Wiley and Sons.

Bower, S. L., Sharrett, M. K., and Plogsted, S. (2006). *Celiac disease—Living with gluten intolerance.* New York: Demos Medical Publishing.

Catassi, C., and Fasano, A. (2008). Is this really celiac disease? Pitfalls in diagnosis. *Current Gastroenterology Reports* 10:466-72.

Haddad, F. G., Maalouly, G., Fahed, J. I., Jammal, M. H., and El Nemnoum, R. J. (2009). Restless leg syndrome in a patient with celiac disease. *Annals of Saudi Medicine* 29(3):238-9.

Häuser, W., Janke, K. H., Klump, B., Gregor, M., and Hinz, A. (2010). Anxiety and depression in adult patients with celiac disease on a gluten-free diet. *World Journal of Gastroenterology* 16:2780-7.

Ratner, A. (2010). Should I worry about gluten in drugs? *Gluten-Free Living,* No. 2, p. 58.

Sarno, J. (2010). When belly troubles don't subside. *Gluten Intolerance Group Magazine* 33: 4, 6, 23.

Sugai, S., Moreno, M. L., Hwang, H. J., Cabanne, A., et al. (2010). Celiac disease serology in patients with different pretest probabilities: Is biopsy avoidable? *World Journal of Gastroenterology* 16:3144-52.

Support groups give seals of approval. (2009). *Gluten-Free Living,* No. 3, p. 29.

Chapter 11

Blumer, I., and Crowe, S. (2010). *Celiac disease for dummies.* New York: John Wiley and Sons.

Bongiobanni, T. R., Clark, A. L., Garnett, E. A., Wojcicki, J. M., Heyman, M. B. (2010). Impact of gluten-free camp on quality of life of children and adolescents with celiac disease. *Pediatrics* 125(3):e525-9.

Buzby, M. (2010). Celiac disease: The endocrine connection. *Journal of Pediatric Nursing* 25:311-3.

Hill, I. D., Dirks, M. H., Liptak, G. S., Colletti, R. B., et al. (2005). Guideline for the diagnosis and treatment of celiac disease in children: Recommendations of the North American Society for Pediatric Gastroenterology, Hepatology and Nutrition. *Journal of Pediatric Gastroenterology and Nutrition* 40:1-19.

James, M. W., and Scott, B. B. (2000). Endomysial antibody in the diagnosis and management of coeliac disease. *Postgraduate Medical Journal* 76:466-8.

Korn, D. (2005). *Venturing out of the house: Restaurant realities.* http://www.celiac.com/articles/864/1/Venturing-Out-of-the-House-Restaurant-Realities-by-Danna-Korn/Page1.html (accessed January 12, 2011).

Mazor, E. (2010). School lunches: How to keep your kids happy and healthy. *Gluten-Free Living,* No. 3, pp. 26, 27.

Moccia, M., Pellecchia, M. T., Erro, R., Zingone, F., et al. (2010). Restless legs syndrome is a common feature of adult celiac disease. *Movement Disorders* 25:877–81.

Ratner, A. (2010). Gluten in gum. *Gluten-Free Living,* No. 3, pp. 30, 31.

Silano, M., Agostoni, C., and Guandalini, S. (2010). Effect of the timing of gluten introduction on the development of celiac disease. *World Journal of Gastroenterology* 16:1939–42.

Chapter 13

Baxter, A. (2010). *Gluten-free travel to Nassau, Bahamas.* http://www.celiac.com/articles/22166/1/Gluten-Free-Travel-to-Nassau-Bahamas/Page1.html (accessed December 27, 2010).

Stone, D. (2010). *Gluten-free camping.* http://www.celiac.com/articles/22128/1/Gluten-Free-Camping/Page1.html (accessed December 27, 2010).

Index